Aging with HIV

Aging with HIV

A Gay Man's Guide

James Masten, Ph.D., LCSW
with James Schmidtberger, M.D.

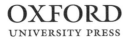

OXFORD
UNIVERSITY PRESS

OXFORD
UNIVERSITY PRESS

Oxford University Press, Inc., publishes works that further
Oxford University's objective of excellence
in research, scholarship, and education.

Oxford New York
Auckland   Cape Town   Dar es Salaam   Hong Kong   Karachi
Kuala Lumpur   Madrid   Melbourne   Mexico City   Nairobi
New Delhi   Shanghai   Taipei   Toronto

With offices in
Argentina   Austria   Brazil   Chile   Czech Republic   France   Greece
Guatemala   Hungary   Italy   Japan   Poland   Portugal   Singapore
South Korea   Switzerland   Thailand   Turkey   Ukraine   Vietnam

Published by Oxford University Press, Inc.
198 Madison Avenue, New York, New York 10016
www.oup.com

Oxford is a registered trademark of Oxford University Press

Library of Congress Cataloging-in-Publication Data

Masten, James.
   Aging with HIV : a gay man's guide / James Masten, with James Schmidtberger.
      p. cm.
   Includes bibliographical references and index.
   ISBN 978-0-19-974058-1 (pbk. : alk. paper)   1. HIV-positive gay men.   2. Older gay men—Health
and hygiene.   3. Older gay men—Psychology.   I. Schmidtberger, James. II. Title.
   RC606.64.M37 2011
   362.196'97920086642—dc22

                                                                    2010023175

ISBN: 978-0-19-974058-1

1 3 5 7 9 8 6 4 2
Printed in the United States of America
on acid-free paper

Disclaimer

The information in this book is not intended to substitute in any way for the health care advice from a trained professional. All health matters, including highly personal ones such as sexual practices and recreational drug use, require medical supervision. This book is a supplement to, but not a replacement for, medical advice on any and all health concerns.

   This book is designed for educational purposes only and should not be used in any other manner. The information contained in this book, including medical screening, testing, and treatments, such as medications, is general in nature and is intended for use as an educational aid only. The information about medications does not cover all possible uses, indications, contraindications, actions, interactions, precautions, or side effects and is not intended as medical advice for individual problems or for making an evaluation as to the risks and benefits of taking a particular medication.

   This book is not intended to substitute for informed medical advice. Advances in medicine may cause information contained here to become outdated, invalid, or subject to debate. You should not use this information to make decisions to screen for, diagnose, or treat a health condition or disease without consulting with a qualified health care provider. Always consult your health care provider with any questions or concerns you may have regarding your health and condition(s). You should always speak with your physician or other health care professional before taking any medication or nutritional, herbal, or homeopathic supplement, before beginning an exercise program, before adopting a health regimen, or before adopting any treatment for a health problem.

   Dr. Schmidtberger's contribution to the book is his own work. His employer, Health and Hospitals Corporation, is not responsible for the content or opinions expressed. You agree to hold harmless the authors, their employers, and the publisher from any and all liability arising directly or indirectly from your use of information contained or referenced in the book, including resources such as other books, websites, support groups, or service organizations. The listings of resources (including, but not limited to, other books, websites, and service organizations) do not constitute an endorsement of that resource, the information, recommendations, or exercises contained therein. You expressly acknowledge and agree that the authors, their employers, and the publishers are not responsible for any consequences of your decisions resulting directly or indirectly from the use of the book.

In memory of Dr. Robert Moore and Roger Kraut

Preface

Between the summer of 2004 and the spring of 2006, I met 15 gay men living with HIV at midlife. I interviewed each one several times, and during the process, I learned a great deal about what it means to age with HIV. The findings from this in-depth qualitative research study earned me a John A. Hartford Doctoral Fellowship and a Ph.D. from New York University School of Social Work. More importantly, however, this experience taught me to reconsider my assumptions about being gay, what it means to live with HIV, and it also caused me to reshape my understanding of aging. What I learned was sometimes surprising, and it was the impetus for writing this book.

I decided that the best way to honor the men who opened up their lives to me, who shared their experience, and built with me a vision of aging with HIV was to tell their stories to help others. Like you, these men are pioneers in the uncharted territory of aging with HIV.

Aging with HIV: A Gay Man's Guide explores the experience of 15 middle-aged gay men living with HIV. It shows how they are managing both the "normal" transitions associated with aging and the additional challenges posed by aging with HIV. The focus of the book is on adaptation, how these men are adapting to aging, what pitfalls they identify, and how you can age successfully while living with the virus.

Is This Book for You?

- Have you lived with HIV longer than you ever expected to?
- Have you spent the past 5, 10, or 20 years dealing with the impact of HIV on your life, your friends, and your community?
- Do you wonder whether changes in your body are due to AIDS or age?
- Have you made plans for your future?
- Are you satisfied with your life today?

If you're like the men with whom I spoke, you probably didn't think you would live long enough to concern yourself with aging. All of a sudden you've become aware of changes in the way you feel physically, in the way others treat you, and in your interests and priorities. Aging with HIV means adapting to a whole list of unexpected changes.

See if you relate to these gay men as they talk about aging with HIV:

Tim[1]:   I never thought I would live this long. I've buried all my friends. I didn't think I'd see forty, and I'm over fifty!

Mario: Now I, pardon my Armenian, I don't give a flying fuck, you know? I just don't care. So I find that the older I've been getting and my friends my own age say the same thing, most of us, you just get to a point where you realize life really just isn't about anything that anybody else thinks. It's about you. It's about what you think. You know and who cares what anyone else thinks?

Luis: Because I don't think of the virus has ... has changed me. I think what's changed me is my age. My wisdom. My experiences. Times. I don't think it's been the virus. I don't think the virus has slowed me down. I think I've slowed down. I'm seeing life different. Because of being a middle aged man. Not because I'm a gay man, or because I'm an HIV man. Because I'm a middle aged man. And I see life and I see people and I see the times and I see how things have changed.

Peter: Bette Davis had it right, "Getting old ain't for sissies."

If you identify with these statements, then consider this: Research on aging tells us that, in general, we follow a somewhat predictable path of development from childhood to old age. Each era of life presents a series of challenges that, when mastered, help us prepare for the next stage of life. In middle adulthood we deal with common issues in the areas of physical changes, career issues, family, and relationships that help us plan for the future. We make decisions such as whether to take a job in a new city, how to care for aging parents, and when to make commitments in our relationships. We travel on this path of development with a cohort of peers who are involved in many of the same tasks. Our peers are not only friends we can rely on for support, they also serve as mirrors of our experience. We compare ourselves to others in our age group to evaluate how we are progressing along our life course.

But AIDS has knocked many gay men off their life course. As Mark put it, *"We are the generation wiped out by HIV."* Since AIDS was first identified in 1981, gay men have been engaged in a consuming battle with HIV. Just as a country at war diverts its resources from areas such as health care to military funding, gay men of this generation have put their efforts into fighting the effects of HIV and AIDS in their bodies and communities.

Meanwhile time has rolled on and aging has affected all the areas of your life: Your body has changed; your friendships and social life are no longer the same, you have a different perspective on work and money, you have a new role in your family, and you have a new attitude about sex and dating. The strategies that you had been using to cope with the challenges of life no longer work in the same way. Whether you recently learned your status or you've been living with HIV for decades, you need help getting back on your life course to make the most of this phase of your life and to prepare for the future.

That's where this book comes in.

How Will This Book Help?

Based on my interviews with gay men living with HIV, research in the fields of aging and HIV, and over 20 years of clinical experience

I have developed a three-part model for optimal aging with HIV: *Changes, challenges*, and *strategies for optimal aging with HIV*.

In Section I, you will identify the nine *changes* common to gay men as they age with HIV, and evaluate how you have adapted to these changes. In Section II, you will see the four *challenges* of aging with HIV, and assess whether you have gotten stuck in the process. And in Section III you will learn ten *strategies* to help you create a path toward optimal aging with HIV.

Included in the ten strategies to optimal aging with HIV is a chapter written by James Schmidtberger, M.D. Although there has been little research on the effects of HIV and its treatments on aging bodies, Dr. Schmidtberger presents the medical knowledge in this area and what you can do to improve your physical health as you age with HIV.

Three categories of text boxes are included in each chapter.

Two types of research boxes will introduce concepts from the fields of gerontology, HIV, gay aging, and mental health. Fast Fact boxes will provide a snapshot of related information.

For example:

FAST FACT

Rates of HIV infection in the United States are experiencing the greatest increase among those in the 50- to 64-year-old age group,[2] and of the 1 million estimated people living with HIV in 2007, 31% were age 50 or older. Given the rate of increase (2.2%) in this group, people over age 50 may represent as much as 40% of those living with HIV in 2010.[3]

Research Review boxes will explain the science behind the topic, giving you a crash course in psychology and physiology, to help you better understand your mind and body and to better communicate with your health care professionals.

Reflection boxes include questions to help you examine how aging has affected your life, evaluate how you are adapting, and identify ways to improve your overall quality of life. You can think about these questions, write out your answers, talk about them with someone else, or work on them in a group.

Finally, each chapter will end with an exercise box with an assignment to complete, and a list of resources available in the community or on the web to further your exploration and provide additional help on the topic.

You can expect to work hard at times. Some sections may be more emotionally challenging for you. It is important that you respect your feelings. It may be necessary to put the book aside for a while if you are feeling vulnerable, tired, sad, or anxious. I will make suggestions when I believe additional support might be helpful. If you have significant changes in your mood such as anger, depression, and anxiety, or if you experience behavioral changes, such as overeating, drinking in excess or other compulsive behaviors, increased isolation or changes in your sleep patterns consult your doctor or psychotherapist. Pace yourself, and seek help from friends or professionals as you see fit.

But you should have fun too. As Patrick pointed out to me, *"Sometimes I just gotta laugh. One thing that aging with this virus has taught me is you've got to have a sense of humor."*

Using This Book in a Group

Group work has been a rite of passage for people living with HIV.[4] Short-term groups have been found to be particularly useful for middle-aged and older people to enhance coping strategies for living with HIV.[5] You can use *Aging with HIV: A Gay Man's Guide* as the foundation for a professionally led or peer facilitated support group. A short-term group using the exercises and activities from this book as a foundation may help individuals reassess and reevaluate their lives in a context of peer support and mutual aid. See page 221 for an outline for using the material in this book in your group.

Are the Concepts in *Aging with HIV: A Gay Man's Guide* Based on Scientific Research?

The changes, challenges, and strategies for optimal aging presented in this book are based, in part, on a research study conducted at

New York University School of Social Work and funded by a fellowship from the John A. Hartford Doctoral Fellows program. The book's contents are also informed by the literature on aging and HIV and by my and Dr. Schmidtberger's decades of clinical practice in the field.

The qualitative research study "Aging with HIV/AIDS: The Experience of Gay Men in Late Middle Age"[6] used a grounded theory methodology to understand the experience of aging with HIV in a group of gay-identified men between the ages of 50 and 65.

Although qualitative research is scholarly in nature and provides important data, there are limitations to this type of study. For example, results from qualitative research are not generalizable to larger populations and cannot provide any suggestions for causal linkage or statistical associations. The study's conclusions were drawn from a small sample of self-selecting participants from the New York City area and the findings may not be applicable to all readers. A full description of the study's methodology and limitations is included in the appendix.

The field of HIV over 50 is a new and expanding area of scientific study. The concept of aging with HIV is a recent development and research on the phenomenon is constantly evolving. Although this book attempts to integrate the most recent findings into a user-friendly format, new developments since the publication of the book may contradict findings presented in this book. It is best to use this guide as a starting point from which you can gather additional data from the resources presented within and from your personal physician in regard to your specific concerns.

On Your Way

Aging with HIV: A Gay Man's Guide will be your guide through the complex changes and challenges that accompany aging with HIV. It is intended to be a helpful tool as you define what successful aging means to you. Keep it handy. You will want to refer to it often as you negotiate the process of aging with HIV.

Acknowledgments

This book is the culmination of several years' work and many colleagues, friends, and family members have contributed to its evolution along the way. Thank you Bridgette Vidunas, Erica Meinhardt, Martha Crawford, Joan Zimmerman, Patricia Grossman, Susannah Moran, Carol Ghiglieri, Ladd Speigel, Curtis Cole, Allison Schachter, Jay Kidd, and Arlene Kochman for your professional guidance, critical readings, and emotional support.

I am grateful to Maura Roessner, my editor, and the staff at Oxford University Press for creating a home for this book and nurturing its development.

To my advisors, Dr. Martha Gabriel, Dr. Robert Moore, Dr. Diane Grodney, and Dr. Cynthia Poindexter—you encouraged me to push past my perceived limitations. And much appreciation goes to Dr. Lubben, Dr. Dunkle, and The John A. Hartford Doctoral Fellows Program for their support.

Thank you, Len and Andrée Pilaro, for strengthening me.

Special thanks go to my parents, Cecele and Irving, my aunt Paulette, my sister Ann, and nephew James.

Thank you to the men who participated in the study and let me into their lives.

And, to my husband, James, much love. I appreciate your enduring support as we brought this work to life. What's next?

Contents

Section I   Aging Means Changing

Introduction   5

Chapter 1   "I'm Still Here."   7

Chapter 2   Physical Changes: AIDS or Age?   16

Chapter 3   Who Do You Consider a Friend
Nowadays?   30

Chapter 4   Being Gay at Midlife   38

Chapter 5   Let's Talk About Sex   47

Chapter 6   Love and Marriage   56

Chapter 7   In the Family   65

Chapter 8   What About Work?   76

Chapter 9   My, How You've Grown   83

Summary   95

Section II   Adaptation versus Stagnation

Introduction   *99*

Chapter 10   Learning from the Past or Living in
the Past?   *102*

Chapter 11   Living within Limitations or Letting
Your World Shrink?   *108*

Chapter 12   Accepting Yourself or Stuck in
Your Ways?   *117*

Chapter 13   One Day at a Time or Avoiding
the Future?   *123*

Summary   *130*

Section III   Ten Steps to Optimal Aging with HIV

Introduction   *135*

Step 1   Care for Your Physical Health   *137*

Step 2   Rebuild and Maintain Your
Social Networks   *149*

Step 3   Be Generative   *157*

Step 4   Fight the Triple Threat: AIDS Stigma,
Homophobia, and Ageism   *161*

Step 5   Let Yourself Grieve   *169*

Step 6   Check Your Baggage   *175*

Step 7   Develop Effective Coping Strategies   *183*

Step 8   Renew Your Spirituality   *189*

Step 9   Plan for the Future   *194*

Step 10   Play   *203*

Conclusion   *207*

About the Study   *209*

Using This Book in a Group   *221*

Notes   *225*

Index   *241*

Aging with HIV

SECTION I
AGING MEANS CHANGING

Introduction

The first step toward optimal aging with HIV is recognizing that aging means changing. In this section you will identify the nine changes common to aging with HIV at midlife, and evaluate how you have been adapting to those changes.

RESEARCH REVIEW

In the study on "Aging with HIV/AIDS: The Experience of Gay Men in Late Middle Age," I conducted in-depth interviews with 15 men living with HIV over the course of 18 months. Through qualitative analysis I found that gay men aging with HIV/AIDS through middle age are encountering a myriad of internal and external changes to which they must adjust, including:

- redefining being gay
- the course of the HIV/AIDS epidemic
- changing friendship networks
- new roles in the family
- changing sex lives and relationships
- a new relationship to productivity
- changing bodies
- and internal changes

These "fields of change," as I refer to them, are both similar to and different from those of other age groups living with

---

HIV/AIDS, HIV-negative gay men at middle age, and aging in the general population. What is different, however, is the unique constellation of changes faced by these men, and the way AIDS diagnosis, caring for others, the magnitude of loss, and the threat of mortality have the potential to inhibit successful adaptation to these changes.[1]

The nine chapters of this section (sex and relationships have been divided into two chapters) parallel the eight axial codes found in my research.

This section of the book is about self-exploration. In it you will review these common changes and evaluate how you have adapted to each change. Seeing where you have come from and how you have traversed these changes will assist you as you move on to the *challenges* to, and *strategies* for, optimal aging with HIV.

Review and reflection are integral aspects of healthy aging. As Joe and Mark point out, reassessment is an important part of defining a new approach to life with HIV at midlife:

> Joe: And from there on, there was a double change that I had to go through. Not only the aging because ... or the middle age business of going from the young person to a middle aged person, but also acquiring a whole new approach to life.
> Mark: It was, you know, it was the right thing to do to take advantage of a new chapter and write something different.

The first change you will review is the course of the epidemic and how you've adapted to the progression of HIV from a terminal illness to a chronic condition.

1

"I'm Still Here."

When I asked Mario about his experience aging with HIV he told me about dealing with the trauma of diagnosis, thinking he was going to die of AIDS, managing opportunistic infections, and losing his closest friends. And then he sang, "I'm still here!" In this song from Steven Sondheim's *Follies* a former starlet turned survivor describes her trials and tribulations, repeatedly concluding that *she's still here.*[1] The song could be an anthem for gay men who have lived into midlife with HIV.

The HIV epidemic is a changing landscape. Once a death sentence, in the developed world HIV has now become a chronic condition. Of course there is reason to celebrate this achievement of modern medicine. But adapting to the changing course of the epidemic has not been easy. First, you had to adjust to life with HIV, the stigma of the disease, and the threat of mortality. Now, you have to adapt to the reality of aging with the disease.

You have been through a lot and are "still here." The first chapter will help you review how you have adapted to the changing course of HIV.

Adjusting to Diagnosis

Mario is a 53-year-old gay man living with AIDS. He was diagnosed in 1992. For him, dealing with the trauma of being diagnosed was the first step in adapting to HIV:

7

You know, it was like getting hit with a brick wall. It really was. It was pretty traumatic to be perfectly honest. It was one of the worst traumas, if not the worst trauma. … I literally walked around shell shocked for about two or three weeks after that. You know, I mean literally.

Perhaps you can relate to Mario's description. For many gay men, even those who thought they might be HIV positive, learning that they have HIV created a shock wave that unsettled every part of their life. After diagnosis most people go through a crisis period, including heightened emotions of depression and anxiety, or numbness. This is a good time to mobilize your resources: to get into counseling, to join an HIV support group or organization, and to seek the support of friends or family.

The initial shock should be short lived as one accepts and adjusts to their status. After living with HIV for almost nine years, Peter is out of the crisis phase:

It becomes conversational. I've now accepted my status, and I'm not as traumatized as I was, certainly.

After living with HIV since 1987, as far as he knows, 54-year-old Mark has integrated HIV into his daily life. Although HIV was once foremost in his thoughts, it is now just a part of him:

I mean I've kind of accepted my HIV status as kind of, you know this is part of my life. This is just so … it's a part of my life. My HIV status, which is positive, is part of my life. And how do I live with it is really the focus.

If You Recently Became Aware of Your HIV Status

Adjusting to being HIV positive can be a challenge at any age. In midlife there are particular issues to face. Joe describes how learning his status at middle age was like a double whammy:

And it, from there on, it … it … there was a double change that I had to go through. Not only the aging because … or the middle age business of going from the young person to a middle aged person, but also acquiring a whole new approach to life.

For many gay men, seroconverting in midlife can add additional stigma. Some men fear judgment from other gay men and have experienced criticism that they "should have known better." Whether you hear that kind of thing from others or not, it is common at any age for people to blame themselves when they contract HIV; that's part of the stigma.

The first thing to do is to reach out to others. In section III you will find resources on where to go for information and support.

For some the trauma of diagnosis lasts longer and the feelings of crisis, fear and depression continue. Clinicians and researchers are examining what makes some people resilient to crisis while others continue to experience trauma long after the event. We know that people who experienced traumas in their past, who have other physical and mental health issues, people who isolate or have little support from friends and family, and people that utilize maladaptive coping strategies, such as relying on alcohol or drugs, may experience greater difficulty adapting to the trauma of HIV. If you have been diagnosed for more than six months and continue to experience symptoms such as frequent crying, panic attacks, nightmares, or flashbacks, lack of interest in activities, or isolation, this is related to trauma and you should speak to a doctor, psychotherapist, or counselor.

REFLECTION

How did you deal with your diagnosis?

People: Who did you rely on?
Places: Where did you go for help?
Activities: What did you do to cope?

Of those people, places, and activities, which are still in your life today?

Living Longer Than Expected

For many gay men who were diagnosed earlier in the epidemic, the next challenge after diagnosis was to manage the threat of major illness and mortality. Most of the gay men I interviewed never thought they would live to midlife. Tim, diagnosed in 1989, put it this way:

> Hopefully I can talk without becoming too emotional. Because all my friends are dead and I just didn't think I would see 40. And I'm 50.

Patrick, a 55-year-old man, diagnosed in 1987, has survived opportunistic infections, bouts of illness, and hospitalizations. He recalls a time when just getting out of bed was a major accomplishment:

> I know what it's like to have to have your butt wiped for you. I don't ever want to become dependent on someone like that again.

Adjusting to life with the threat of illness and mortality has not been easy. Some of the men describe it as an extra burden that they carry, weighing down their thoughts and feelings and even causing body aches and fatigue.

The second task of living longer than expected is to learn to live with chronic illness. Patrick now believes that his medication regimen has HIV under control. He takes 12 pills a day and has learned to live with chronic conditions including fatigue, weight loss, diarrhea, diabetes, and heart disease. He says that sometimes taking care of his health feels like a full-time job.

Finally, living longer than expected has involved a change in focus from "How *can* I live with HIV?" to "How do I *want* to live?" Mark, a 54-year-old gay man who was diagnosed in 1987, has lived through the trauma of diagnosis, has learned to manage the threat of mortality, and has learned to live with the complications of chronic illness. Recently, he realized that he wants more out of life than to just survive with HIV:

> I mean I've kind of accepted my HIV-status as kind of, you know, this is part of my life. My HIV status, which is positive, is part of my life. And how do I live with it is really the focus.

RESEARCH REVIEW

Davies describes the process of living with HIV as "Struggling first to reduce their projected biographical time and then, after having outlived it, year by year to recreate their future already given up."[2]

Adjustment to chronicity shapes one's sense of self, time, and body[3] and involves coping with physical, financial, psychological, and social losses.[4] It has been found that there is no formula or prescription for coping with the chronicity of HIV/AIDS, but multiple pathways in which well-being can be achieved.[5] Mitchell and Linsk have pointed out the number of new challenges people living with HIV/AIDS face as the disease transitions from a terminal illness to a chronic one. Included in this list are questions about when to initiate medical treatment, how to cope with and manage long-term and still very serious illness, and how to cultivate intimate relationships with minimal fear of passing the virus on or being reinfected.[6]

Adapting to the changing course of the illness can involve developing new attitudes toward information seeking, shifts in involvement with HIV organizations, and reassessment of the effectiveness and appropriateness of HIV support groups. Although the men I interviewed remain involved in HIV organizations and groups, their needs have changed, and, several note, the organizations have not changed with them. For some, this means moving to groups with older members, men whose experience mirrors their own. And for others this change has meant leaving support groups that, as Hector said, "talk about HIV all the time," something, after all these years, he is tired of hearing about.

Groups, once a rite of passage for gay men living with HIV, continue to serve as communities of support for people aging with the virus.[7] Robinson and colleagues document how one support group has evolved in response to the changing course of the illness. As their group members aged with HIV they added older men who recently learned their serostatus. The mixture of their differing approaches and issues enriched the group to become "a context in which members can share very different challenges of aging with HIV, drawing on each others' strengths."[8]

Living with HIV means changing your focus from surviving to thriving. Earlier in your illness you may have made decisions thinking you would not live into middle and older age. These choices included going on disability, moving to be closer to a support network, cashing out insurance policies, etc. Adapting to living longer than you expected involves reviewing those choices, acknowledging the adaptations you have made to live with HIV, and assessing whether those are still applicable today.

REFLECTION

What does it mean to you to live with HIV today?
How often do you think of HIV?
When do those thoughts most often occur?
Do you think that you will die from HIV?
How do you think those thoughts affect your day-to-day life?

Living Through Loss

The changing course of the illness has not only involved adapting to HIV in your body, it has also meant coping with a magnitude of loss. The AIDS epidemic has been a holocaust for gay men, and the men I spoke with had lost most or all of their friends and acquaintances. For Mario, Tim, and Patrick aging with HIV has meant dealing with overwhelming losses:

> Mario: And especially since my friends are dropping dead right and left, you lived with that feeling of, am I next? You know and the feeling that there could have very well been that you could be next.
>
> Tim: I am of the generation that was wiped out by the holocaust. This holocaust happened to be AIDS.
>
> Patrick: But when you can open up your address book and start crossing out names and it gets over a hundred names in your life of people that shouldn't be dead already, clearly something monstrous ... monstrous is happening.

One common reaction to the magnitude of loss is survivor guilt. After losing a partner and many friends to AIDS, Patrick recognizes that he became hardened:

> You know, sometimes I'll remember a friend that I really did love, that I really did care about, and … because the losses were coming so rapidly and so, wave after wave after wave, I didn't … I argued myself out of loving those people. I managed to convince myself that they weren't that important in order to keep going, you know? I think I feel a lot of guilt. I mean one thing, I was thinking this before you came today and I thought, well, we have to say this out loud, even if we don't necessarily have to explore it or talk about it or elaborate on it, but like people in the holocaust, there's survivors' guilt that plays out in my life is … when I talk about Philip being dead and Roger being dead, then I feel it's like, well [Patrick], you're not.

Mark and Hector are trying to learn from their losses:

> Mark: So in retrospect, what did you get out of that? You lost someone you loved dearly, but what did you learn from it? I learned the beauty of that individual. I learned parts of that person that I want to be, you know? And I also learned the parts of that person I don't want to be.
>
> Hector: So I'm figuring it's gotta be a reason why I'm still alive. See we're all here for a purpose. We don't know that purpose but …

It is easy to become mired in the grief of multiple losses. This can lead to survivor guilt, hopelessness, and depression. Someone mired in loss is apathetic to life, has little energy to devote to self-care, and has no interest in planning for the future.

It is equally compelling to avoid loss, allow numbness to take over, and deny any feelings of grief. Although this approach can seem to alleviate the pain, if you deny feelings of loss you can become cut off from all your feelings, from other gay men, and, ultimately, from your passion for life and reason for living.

> **FAST FACT**
>
> Resilience in the wake of multiple losses to AIDS involves:
>
> - living in a way that does not deny loss
> - without feeling consumed by grief[9]

Becoming resilient in the face of multiple losses and allowing yourself to mourn without becoming consumed with grief are significant parts of adapting to the changing course of the epidemic. Remember, *grieving gives honor to both the lives of those that have died and to your own life.*

REFLECTION

How are you coping with loss?
Do you avoid thinking about friends who have died?
Do you feel guilty for being alive?
Do you feel overwhelmed by grief?
What do you do to honor those losses and to learn from them?

HIV: From a Terminal Illness to a Chronic Condition

The first change that you have managed while aging with HIV is a complex one. Adjusting to the changing course of the epidemic has involved adapting to the trauma of diagnosis and the threat of mortality, learning to live with the effects of HIV and the medications, and living through devastating losses.

We all need to adapt to the changing course of the illness. During the 1980s and 1990s when my partner, my friends, and my clients were ill and dying of AIDS, I was in a constant "crisis mode." I developed strategies to deal with the stress. As the disease progression changed, I had to alter my approach, both personally and professionally. Crisis intervention was no longer the most appropriate modality in either area. I had to develop the ability to think long term. Writing this book is part of that process for me.

■ **ASSIGNMENT** ■

Make a dream list. What would you like to do? Travel, work, relationships, etc. Let yourself go. Write everything down, no matter how outlandish it seems.

(Maybe you always wanted to become a real estate tycoon, to play the drums, to travel the world, or to write a self-help book?)

Only after you have written every fantasy down can you review the list. Is there anything on that list that is surprising? Anything that you forgot about or gave up on?

Find one thing on that list that you can start to work toward today. What can you do to reach that goal?

In this chapter you have reflected on the changing course of the epidemic and reviewed the adaptations you have made along the way. Ultimately, adapting to aging with HIV today involves rediscovering how you want to live your life and planning for a newly rediscovered future. In the third section of the book I will outline 10 *strategies* for optimal aging with HIV to help you in that process. In the next chapter you will examine how aging with HIV has changed your body.

2

Physical Changes: AIDS or Age?

We all know that our bodies change as we age, yet accepting those changes is another matter. Ronald recalls how hard it was for him to accept those physical changes:

I used to play basketball with some fellows I worked with …
and I came home and my back would hurt so bad I could
hardly move … Well, after the third time, I realized, I just
can't play basketball with those young guys anymore.

It took a few days of being laid up in bed with a heating pad for Ronald to accept that he could no longer play basketball as he used to. But eventually he adapted and adjusted his lifestyle. He has since joined a gym and is thinking about finding a new group of guys closer to his age to play with.

The process of acceptance of and adaptation to a changing body is more complex when you are aging with HIV. Fluctuations in HIV-related symptoms, complications from the medication, and the question of whether physical changes are age or AIDS can make it difficult to know what choice is best. This chapter will help you review how you have adapted to your changing body.

HIV-Related Changes

If you are like the men I interviewed, you continue to experience HIV-related changes. You have learned to live with fluctuating symptoms, such as fatigue, nausea, body aches, neuropathy, and diarrhea.

Luis says that HIV barely interferes with his life. He explains,

There are times when I'm really tired. I get these skin irritations at times. I was told by the nurse that was HIV-related. That's all.

In fact, adapting to HIV-related symptoms today may seem like nothing compared to the challenges faced in the early days of the epidemic. In the 1980s George wasn't sure whether he was going to live or die. He had been hospitalized several times and needed home health care to help him with basic tasks such as eating, bathing himself, and going to the bathroom. When he compares his current health to the past he barely notices his HIV-related symptoms.

Mario finds that adapting to his HIV-related physical changes is manageable:

It's tiredness, weakness ... pains here and there in the muscles. Occasional bouts of peripheral neuropathy but not too bad ... it's all handleable.

For Arthur, a new challenge arose when, after living with HIV with no symptoms for many years, his T cell count began dropping and his doctor recommended antiviral treatment:

I have to also learn to accept a lot of things. And I cannot. I have to evolve. Well, you know I am no longer ... Well, things have changed that I now have to take a cocktail, uh, and I just accept it and it's another form of evolution. And that evolution is, because of accepting that and realizing that it is, that there's no such thing as immortality, and I'm embracing life as it is and challenging myself.

RESEARCH REVIEW
HIV AND AGING: WHAT WE KNOW

Middle aged and older people:

- Are undertested for HIV
- Are at increased risk of opportunistic infections and complications with delayed diagnosis[1]

- Had more rapid progression toward AIDS and death before the era of highly active antiretroviral therapy (HAART)
- May have delayed immune recovery in the HAART era[2]
- Demonstrate a higher risk of excess mortality[3,4]

There are few studies examining treatment outcomes in middle-aged and older adults and no age-specific guidelines for the use of antiviral medications in this group. What we do know is that:

- Older adults have better adherence to treatment regimens and are less likely to interrupt antiviral treatment[5,6]
- Antiviral therapy suppresses HIV as well in older adults as other groups
- Younger adults' CD4 cell counts appear to rebound more quickly and higher than older adults'[7]
- Despite viral suppression, older adults may have a higher risk of clinical progression to an AIDS-defining illness
- Rates of treatment regimen changes due to toxicity appear higher in older adults; due to age-related decreases in kidney function and liver function, there is decreased medication clearance from the body, increased drug levels in the blood, and increased side effects[8]

Several "comorbid conditions" (health conditions or diseases present in your body at the same time) concern middle-aged and older individuals living with HIV at a greater rate,[9] including:

- Osteoporosis and bone disease
- Cardiovascular disease*
- Impaired fasting glucose ("prediabetes")
- Diabetes

- Increased cholesterol
- Body fat composition changes (lipoatrophy and lipohypertrophy)
- Neurocognitive dysfunction
- Non-AIDS-defining cancers

*HIV-infected people appear to have an increased cardiovascular risk compared to uninfected counterparts, yet this risk may be due to antiviral therapy, HIV itself, or both. Although there is evidence that antiviral treatment raises risk factors (e.g., increased high blood pressure, cholesterol, and prediabetes), recent studies have also found that antiviral treatment may, in fact, reduce these risk factors. At this time, the benefits of treatment clearly outweigh the risks. Current recommendations are to reduce modifiable risk factors (including obesity, smoking, and a sedentary lifestyle) and treat high blood pressure and cholesterol abnormalities.

HIV Care

Although there is no one strategy for adapting to HIV-related physical changes, several of the men I talked to said that it is important to prioritize your health care. Maintaining a regular self-care regimen is a way to commit to yourself and your body. Joe makes sure he meditates and takes a walk every day. He also goes to the gym regularly, does not drink, smoke, or take drugs, eats sensibly, and takes vitamins and herbal treatments.

Mario believes that modifying his use of drugs and alcohol is one of the key factors in his survival with HIV:

> But I think that my instincts were good in knowing enough to stop all the drugs and everything that I was using in my youth. That my instincts of self-preservation kicked in and it may or may not be true but I tend to think it is true that I'm the living proof.

FAST FACT

Not only has excessive drug and alcohol use been associated with HIV disease progression,[10] but in the study of adult development, alcohol abuse and heavy smoking are two of the six values measured at age 50 that best predict illness and mortality by age 75.[11] The use of drugs, tobacco, and alcohol will be discussed in greater depth in the Steps to Optimal Aging.

Mark places importance on stress reduction:

You should be thinking about your physical health. You should get some exercise or you should be doing things to reduce your stress level or learning how to breathe and eating well, whatever. Your mental health. Feeling good about what you're doing.

Everyone has his own health care strategy. Tim pushes himself through fatigue:

I have difficulty accepting that I have to slow down. I still try to multitask but it doesn't work anymore. I have a much shorter fuse. I get spent quicker than I normally do. And taking that nap to me is accepting defeat.

Although Mario lets himself rest when he needs to:

My m.o. is that if I can hike myself out of bed, up to the mirror, and make myself presentable then I can go to work. And now it just doesn't work, because even if I can do that, I still have to go back to bed.

Keeping up with a regimen after years of caring for your health can be exhausting, and sometimes you just want to take a break. Here is what some of the guys say about caring for their health when you have HIV:

Patrick: If you get the flu that's a horrible thing. But, if you get the flu and you're HIV positive, does it mean you might be in store for some other things?

Could you be open to opportunistic infections that you thought were history, but that might come back now, because you got sick? So, that constant sense of involvement in my own health is exhausting.

Peter: It worries me, not overly worries me. I feel as though I'm getting, a little, uh, lax, with wanting to go and do blood work, on top of that. It's almost like I've done it. Having dealt with it for as many years, five or six years now, and, uh, I don't know, I've gotten a little phobic about it, going back and checking up and making sure that everything is okay. That's a strange assumption that everything is okay, or that everything will be okay too. That's, uh, kind of like disavowing of reality, like, too. I'm HIV positive now so, uh, I'll get around to it. You know what it's doing—it's a distraction technique for me to sort of keep myself on hold, a little bit in limbo. Cause things are going so incredibly well.

Arthur: I'm not a number person. I feel good and I look good, that's all that matters. I'm going to keep myself with numbers, it's gonna drive you crazy, stress you out. I have friends that have one T cell. I've gotten to the point where I don't think about numbers anymore.

George has lived with HIV for 20 years. He regularly visits a physician, a cardiologist, an ophthalmologist, a physical therapist, a nutritionist, a chiropractor, an acupuncturist, and a psychotherapist. Sometimes George feels he has had enough:

I go to the doctors an awful lot. [lists doctors] Enough doctors! There are weeks when I see doctors practically all the time, every day. How could you have a full time job going to so many doctors? You couldn't.

Jamie, however, welcomes the deepening relationship he has formed with his doctor over the years:

I was worried that they were going to send me a letter that I was going to the doctor too much, so I started to slow down, because I used to go to the doctor every week. And we used to sit down and talk. Because her and I, I don't know how to explain the relationship, but we can really talk to each other. We don't have to pull no punches with each other.

In Section III we will discuss in more depth how you can partner with your doctor and build a health care regimen that is both manageable and flexible, and takes into consideration changes in your health over time. The key is not to commit to something that feels too cumbersome or you are likely to give up altogether.

Take a moment now to reflect on the adaptations you have made to take care of your HIV-related health.

REFLECTION

What physical changes do you associate with HIV?

How have you adapted your life to deal with these symptoms (such as fatigue or diarrhea)?

Write out your health care regimen (the activities you do on a daily or weekly basis to care for your body).

Now, reevaluate your self-care regimen:

Are there other things you want to be doing to improve your health?

Are there activities that were once helpful, but that can now be put aside?

Medication-Related Changes

Aging is the latest challenge in HIV-related health care in the developed world. Doctors, once focused on keeping people alive, are now treating patients with complications from years of taking HIV medications. Even if you've only just begun taking medications, you may already be noticing side effects. The most common side effects from HIV medications affect the digestive track (i.e., nausea, diarrhea, vomiting, and loose stools). Other symptoms include headache, dizziness and fatigue, neuropathy, and kidney disease. The PDR (*Physicians' Desk Reference*) is filled with side effects from medications and recommendations for use. Sustiva™, for example, can affect your central nervous system and cause a disconnected feeling, so doctors recommend that it be taken at night.[12] Often your body adapts to the medication, and symptoms can go away within days, months, or may never go away.

Doctors are just beginning to understand the long-term effects of taking HIV medications. Research and experience indicate that the long-term effects of taking some of these medications include abnormal weight gain, elevated cholesterol, and diabetes, among others, all of which play a role in heart disease. However, diagnosing the cause of these symptoms is complex. As a case in point, there is emerging research indicating that HIV itself, rather than medication side effects, may be playing a direct role in heart disease (see, for example, Lee, Sharon Dian, *HIV and Aging*, 2008; Informa Healthcare USA, New York, pp 41–53).

Our understanding of HIV and the interactions of medications is always evolving. At one time, if you stayed informed, you could know almost as much as (and sometimes, more than) your doctor about HIV. Now, there is so much information, it is difficult to stay abreast. Luis remembers when he used to seek out the latest HIV information, but now he takes his HIV status for granted:

> 14 years now in September. So you know it's like I'm getting over it. It's like, oh wow, you know? At the beginning, no, it was like oh, everything was HIV. I wanted to read everything HIV. And everything I saw was HIV and I wanted to know as much as I can. Now it's just like, you know it's a daily routine. I pick it up, I get dressed, I take a shower, I go to bed, I eat, that's just with it. That goes along with it.

Remember, you are still a pioneer in the world of aging with HIV and you may find that given the increased complexities, you need to step it up and, once again, become more informed and involved in order to manage your HIV and its treatment at this stage of your life.

Adapting to changes in your body can be further complicated when HIV and its treatment cause disruptions in your physical health. Tim has been taking HIV medications for years, and although his T cell level is high and his viral load remains undetectable, he has occasional fatigue and diarrhea, which he attributes to his medication regimen. Patrick has developed diabetes. As a result he has developed impotence. He sometimes wonders whether it was worth it, but quickly reminds himself that he was near death only a few years ago:

> I think that most of the problems I've encountered have been due to … side effects from the medications. Now who knows what would've happened without the medications? You know that's the choice you make when you decide, OK, I'll take the medication regimen.

FAST FACT

Everything has side effects: the medications you take, the herbal supplements you buy, and the dessert you eat. If you take it in, it has the potential to change your body. Deciding which side effects are acceptable is a choice we make on a daily basis.

Lipodystrophy

Perhaps the most talked about physical change is lipodystrophy. Lipodystrophy is a collection of syndromes: lipohypertrophy, excess fat accumulation where the back and neck meet or inside the abdomen; lipoatrophy, loss of fat in the arms, legs, or cheeks; or an increase in triglycerides, a type of cholesterol. Lipodystrophy can take an emotional toll. Both Mario and Mark referred to their lipodystrophy as "the scarlet A," the sign that declares their HIV status to the world. For Joe it has raised both shame and fear of other people's pity. He talks about how it impacts his involvement in the world:

> Well that's my biggest … it affects my life in, well, on a daily basis and even deep down in, you know, personality. I don't like going out. I don't like … I don't accept invitations to large gatherings, you know? I don't go to any family, you know, kinds of things. This is the appearance of AIDS. That's why. I'm a very private person, and I would prefer to have my privacy all around. So this compromises my privacy.

At one time in your illness you had to deal with the reality of taking medications with severe side effects to combat HIV. And that was a tough pill to swallow. Today, you see the compounding effects of these medications on your body. From inconveniences to major illnesses, you take pills to treat the effects of the pills you have taken for so long. Use the following questions to reflect on your adaptations to medication-related changes.

REFLECTION

List the symptoms that you attribute to the medication you take.

How does this affect your feelings about the medications? Your compliance with taking them? Have you ever discussed this with your doctor?

Do the visible signs of lipodystrophy have an impact on your self-esteem and social involvement?

Have you discussed this with anyone else?

Age-Related Changes

At midlife men begin to experience subtle changes in their body. New aches and pains arise, changes in agility and energy can occur, and visual changes are evident. At 57, Jamie is noticing slight changes in his body:

> Your lower back might hurt you sometimes. There's different pains you get different places that you know you didn't used to get before.

In fact, each of the men I interviewed identified physical changes that they attributed to their age:

> Luis: I'm having senior moments. Forgetting.
> Arthur: Oh maybe when I feel a little sick or I feel a little tired. I say, damn I'm tired. Well, I'm 51 years old.
> Ronald: So the need for eyeglasses or ... or ... or ... or sight aids become necessary. And there are other little telltale signs like that. You begin to slow down and ...

RESEARCH REVIEW

In the general population memory performance and cognitive functions do not change significantly at middle age,[13] and unrecognized hearing loss (evident in a third of men over 65) is often confused with decreased mental functioning.[14]

Although there is some change in cognitive functions found in middle-aged and older people living with HIV, this field of research is still new and currently there is mixed evidence to determine whether advanced age decreases cognitive functioning in this population.[15] There is limited research that has found that people living with HIV have functional brain patterns similar to people 15 years older.[16] For those that demonstrate neurocognitive impairment, it is difficult to determine causality due to age, HIV, long-term medication use, or poorer medication adherence.[17]

Strategies to maintain and increase cognitive functioning will be discussed in Section III.

As we age, medical issues arise that we are prone to because of our family history. Lifestyle, too, plays a significant role in aging. Changeable factors, such as a sedentary lifestyle and smoking, for example, are among the top risk factors for heart disease.

RESEARCH REVIEW

There is no one pattern by which we age. In fact, there is disagreement among researchers about why we age in the first place.[18] However, there are some physical changes that are associated with this stage of life.[19] At midlife we can expect changes in:

- appearance (including skin, hair, and teeth)
- bodily functions (musculoskeletal, respiratory, cardiac, urinary, and digestion)
- sensory function (hearing, sight, taste, and smell)

- nervous system (especially sleep patterns) and
- reproductive and sexual patterns (discussed in Chapter 5)

It is important to distinguish normal aging from disease progression. Some illnesses commonly associated with aging are more often the result of heredity, environment, and life-style. For example, although half of all adults over age 65 have evidence of heart disease, there are significant modifi-able risk factors, including hypertension, diabetes, high cho-lesterol, obesity, alcohol use, smoking, diet, and sedentary lifestyle.

Primarily, adapting to these age-related changes involves making minor adjustments in the way we take care of ourselves—how we eat, exercise, and work. But making these changes means that we have accepted our aging. The longer we resist the effects of aging on our bodies, the harder those challenges can become.

One day while researching this book, I went for a jog and sprained my ankle. Full of the cocky, self-assuredness of young adulthood I didn't see a doctor, pushed through the pain, and it healed. But I find that it's not quite the same as the other ankle.

A couple years later, while writing the book, I injured my shoulder while working out. (Yes, I may be a klutz.) This time, I learned from my mistake. I went to the doctor, who prescribed physical therapy, and my shoulder healed properly.

It was a process for me to accept that my body was aging and that I could no longer ignore my aches and pains until they went away. Appreciating the changes in my aging body allows me to learn how to care for it better.

Age or AIDS?

Often people with HIV have difficulty determining whether symptoms are age- or HIV-related. Symptom ambiguity is a common theme in my interviews, as well as much of the research on HIV in people over 50.[20] Mario talks about his fatigue in this way:

> Also physically, you know? I don't have as much pep as I used to. Whether or not that's my serostat, you know, whether it's HIV or just old age, I don't know. Or if it's a combination of both, which is probably it.

Knowing whether a symptom is related to age or AIDS can affect how you choose to address it. Yet, as you have probably experienced, determining a cause can be difficult for you and your doctor. Hypertension, diabetes, and hypercholesterolemia are all conditions that can be brought out by the interaction of HIV, its medication, family history, and lifestyle.

Questions you should ask yourself include the following: Is this a normal symptom of aging that I should accommodate? Does it suggest a new HIV-related illness that needs to be treated? Is it a complication from the medication? Is it related to lifestyle or depression?

The information your body is giving you is an important gauge to determine how best to care for it.

■ ASSIGNMENT ■

How do you know whether a symptom is age- or HIV-related? Consider the assumptions you make and how they impact your treatment decisions.

Make a list with three columns.
In the first column write down all your physical symptoms.
In the second column write down whether you believe the symptom is caused by HIV, a side effect of the medications, or age.
In the third column write down how you deal with the symptom. Assess whether that approach worked or whether you need to try something else.

Review your second column. Why did you choose each answer? How would you alter your response to the symptom (column 3) if you changed your answer?
Discuss these choices with your doctor.

In this chapter you identified the physical changes that accompany aging with HIV and the difficulty you may sometimes have in distinguishing symptoms as age-related or HIV-related. Keep this review in mind as you proceed through the book. Understanding your physical changes and what you do to accommodate them has implications throughout your life. In the next chapter you will consider how aging with HIV involves adapting to changes in your friendship networks.

3

Who Do You Consider a Friend Nowadays?

> **Mario: Well, I mean I lost virtually all my good friends to AIDS. All my good, gay friends I lost, every one.**

The AIDS epidemic has wiped out a generation of gay men, and left the survivors with decimated friendship networks and social supports. Why, then, do I write a chapter asking gay men at midlife to question who they call a friend? *Because man is a social animal, and we need our friends to survive.* Regardless of the magnitude of your loss, you must rebuild your social networks.

In each era of life our needs and requirements for friendships change. Adding new friends at this stage of your life requires self-examination. This chapter will help you review who you call a friend, and why.

Shared Experiences

A significant part of friendship lies in the bond of shared experiences. With our peers we reminisce about our common past, compare our current experience, as well as give and receive advice, support, and camaraderie with people who understand us. Mario has a few close friends, most of whom are HIV positive. He talks about how important it is for him to have the support of people who are going through the same thing:

> It, well, you know, I do have a bunch of ... there are about three or four people at GMHC that I, you know, consider

friends. It's important to me to be in touch with people. Other people who are going through the same thing and dealing with similar things.

As Joe got older he recognized that he wanted friends closer to his own age:

So I began to need people that were older to share with, because I no longer had that much in common with younger people in that sense.

REFLECTION

Make a list of people you consider friends. What makes these people friends?

What do you have in common?

How often do you contact them? Do you see them or speak on the phone? When was the last time you were in touch with someone on that list?

RESEARCH REVIEW

Building satisfying friendship networks and maintaining a "convoy" of social support are among the most salient features of healthy aging. Having a group of friends with whom one shares the experiences of aging provides a protective layer of social relations to guide, socialize, and encourage individuals as they move through life.[1] For gay men, the concept of a convoy is especially important, and support from friends has been emphasized as an integral tool to combat the experience of homophobia.[2]

Yet people over 50 living with HIV are found to have fragile networks of social support, to be more isolated, and to be less satisfied with their friendship networks.[3] In a study of HIV in people over 50, Schrimshaw and Siegel identified several perceived barriers to obtaining social support, including nondisclosure, others' fear, the desire to be self-reliant, not wanting to be a burden, the unavailability of family, the death of friends to AIDS, and ageism.[4]

Changing Needs

As we change, so does our need for friends. Mario was once into the club scene, and his friends were "guys who knew how to party and have fun." He laughs when he considers how far away he feels from his days of drinking and drugging with a "bunch of bitchy queens." Now he appreciates people to go to the theater and movies with, who he can sit and talk to, and who make him feel good about himself. He talks about the process of making friends today:

> And it's a sifting process. I've, you know, some have come in, and then I realize, wait a minute, I don't want them in. You know … just because you're gay and have AIDS doesn't make you a good person. You know, learned that lesson. So there's a sifting process that goes on. But I have met a lot of nice people and I've met a lot of assholes. But that's life. You know, regardless of status.

If you need different things from a friend than you did when you were younger, then you have to look for friends in different places. George, who lost all of his friends to AIDS, talks about making younger friends who can take care of him as he gets older. Patrick likes having friends from different backgrounds:

> I just thought, you know, I need to have some people in my life who are HIV negative. And straight, maybe.

Recognizing how you have changed is an integral part of evaluating what you want from a friend.

REFLECTION

Now, return to your list. In what ways do people on that list
    differ from you? How many are HIV negative, straight, or
    younger than you?
How have your requirements for friendship changed over the
    years?

Are You Open to New Friendships?

*When I was 8 years old, my family moved to a new neighborhood.
I had lived in the same house for as long as I could remember and my
best friends were my next-door neighbors. In my new house I was
lonely, but I was so anxious about making friends that I stayed inside
when I saw the neighbors playing on the block. Finally, my mother
pushed me out of the house, saying, "You're not going to make new
friends sitting in front of the TV."*

Mom was right. Thinking about making friends didn't accomplish anything, except increase my anxiety. I just had to get out
there. Now, before you dismiss the relevance of this story to your
life, consider Hector. He has lost many friends to AIDS. After being
diagnosed with HIV in his fifties, he has had to rebuild his life. He
wants to make new friends, but rarely goes out of the house. When
asked how he spends his time, he says, "I do get into TV." And
Hector is not alone. Several of the men I spoke with would like to
have more friends, but have not made much effort to do so. Half
the men I interviewed had a pet, and most of them referred to
their pet as an important source of friendship; as Mario said with
a smile, referring to his dog, "This is my significant other." Pets can
be significant sources of support, but they cannot replace people.

The Internet can be a great tool for making new friends. We can
keep in contact with friends across the globe, join chat groups with
like-minded people, and feel connected to others when distance or
illness isolates us. The Internet can be especially helpful for the
homebound or for people in regions in which there are no organizations or groups serving gay, HIV-positive, or older people. For those
who have a tendency toward isolation, however, the Internet can be
used as an excuse to avoid contact with people. Use the Internet as
a supplement to your friendship network, not as a replacement.

RESEARCH REVIEW

This book emerged from the experience of gay men living in New York City. In fact, the majority of research on HIV in people over 50 draws from urban communities. Among people living with HIV, across age groups, research finds that rural people with HIV have a significantly lower satisfaction with life, lower perceptions of social support from family members and friends, reduced access to medical and mental health care, elevated levels of loneliness, more community stigma, heightened personal fear that their HIV serostatus would be learned by others, and more maladaptive coping strategies, such as avoidance or drinking in excess, than those from urban areas.[6] Although telephone-based support groups have been shown to be an effective intervention to reduce barriers to care and provide emotional support for HIV-positive individuals in rural areas, and to improve coping and emotional well-being for older people living with HIV in both rural and urban areas, they are not widely offered.[7]

If you are from a rural community, you have probably developed creative strategies to reach out to other gay, HIV-positive, and older men. Although you may feel all alone out there, remember that you are not the only one and that there are people who understand what you are going through. Keep in contact with people you know, use the telephone, look for new people to whom you can relate in your community, and use the Internet for support.

As you think about who you consider a friend, ask yourself what steps you have taken to make new friends and what, if anything, could be interfering with the process of meeting new people. You may have anxiety about talking to strangers or being rejected. You could have insecurity about what you have to offer, not know how to meet people, and not know where to go. There could be financial or physical obstacles to overcome. For Tim, the challenge of making new friends is dealing with the risk of experiencing more loss:

I think that there are as many people in my life as I can take. Which is different from people that I like. Because the people that I like are all dead. And I think that, I often say this.

The reason that I don't have many people in my life. Very few. And none of them are of the closeness in relationship as any of them were, because the loss was so great. And I'm just afraid of losing them all over again.

For George, the obstacle is money:

It's making the idea of looking for new friends difficult … because what does an interesting person want to do with me who can't do anything?

And Peter simply acknowledges:

I'm not great at establishing friendships and long-term relationships.

Despite all the challenges, Mario keeps trying to make new friends:

I have met new acquaintances and I made a couple of good friends. I lost people that I had been friends with for 30 years. You know, lifelong friends. So these are relatively new friends.

RESEARCH REVIEW

Access to, use of, and satisfaction with friendship networks are key factors for successful aging[8] as well as for health and well-being for middle-aged and older people with HIV.[9] In a study comparing the effect of social support on mood among gay men living with HIV, not only was social support found to mitigate distress and improve affect, but the influence of social support on mood was significantly greater for middle-aged and older gay men with HIV when compared with the younger sample.[10]

The AIDS epidemic has significantly reshaped your circle of friends. But aging, too, involves changes in who you consider a friend. Adapting to aging with HIV means reevaluating what you want from a friend today and what you have done to make new friends.

■ ASSIGNMENT ■

Imagine that there is a corporation whose sole mission is to take care of your well-being, and it is your job to staff the company properly.

My Company

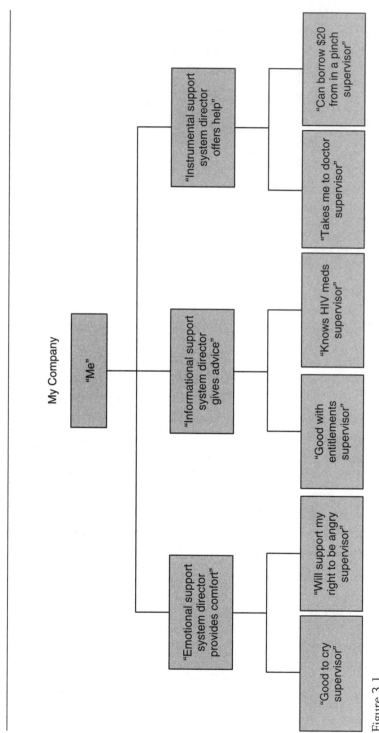

Figure 3.1

First, determine the positions you will need to fill.

What are the company's departments? (The department of emotional support; of smart people with good suggestions; calm people in the face of crisis; mood improvers; people who tell it like it is; transportation services; the department of people who can reach things on the top shelf of the cupboard, etc.)

Draw an organizational chart (Fig. 3.1).

Then see which of those sections are already staffed. How many friends do you have to cover each position? Do some of your "staff" have duties in several areas? Where are there gaps?

Make a recruitment plan. How will you fill those empty positions?

In this chapter you have reviewed how aging with HIV has changed your friendship networks, how your needs for a friend have altered, and what you've done to adapt to these changes. Section III of the book will go into more detail and give suggestions about how to rebuild your friendship networks. In the next chapter you will evaluate how your gay identity has changed as you've been aging with HIV.

4

Being Gay at Midlife

Luis: I remember from the Stonewall. We've come a long a
way because you couldn't hold hands or kiss a guy in
the street the way you can now, or be it so openly, and
all these gay rights, and all these TV shows, we didn't
have that on TV. *Queer as Folk*. When? Who'd ever
thought. I never thought that things like that would
happen. So, it's like getting married. You couldn't walk
the streets together, they would beat you up, now
you're getting married. So, it's a long way we've come.

Being gay has changed dramatically since the pre-Stonewall era.
As Joe says, "It's completely different. Like night and day." And for
the most part these changes are positive. But even changes for the
better involve adjustment, and growing from a young man grap-
pling with identity in a homophobic society to a middle-aged man
living with HIV involves adapting to a great deal of change. This
chapter will help you review your always-evolving sexual identity.

Coming Out

In my work facilitating groups with gay men in midlife the first
topic discussed is usually "coming out." Sharing coming out stories
helps group members bond over their common experience. Telling
these stories breaks the isolation and shame that were once so
much a part of being gay. It may seem that it's been a long time

since you felt like the only one, but those memories have shaped who you are today. See if you identify with Mario's experience of facing stigma:

> Growing up was not easy. It was horrible. It was trauma, it was filled with trauma. I thought I was the only gay person in the world. It was nuts. It took me a long time to get through that.
>
> It was always a waiting game of them finding out that people really didn't want you around because you were gay. I had a couple of instances of that. Where, you know, I'd get hired and then when they realized what was up they made it plain that they didn't want that kind of person around. Things were very different. I mean, I think it probably still happens now. But it was really, you know, that was common.

Today, we know that coming out is not a single event, but a lifelong process that includes subtle choices, such as whose photos you display, what pronouns you use, when and where you hold hands publicly, who you tell, and when you remain silent. Your experience of stigma and coming out impacts how you cope with HIV and aging.

REFLECTION

Remember what life was like for you before you "came out." If you have a photo of yourself then, look at it. Or take a snapshot of yourself in your mind's eye.

Now, look at your face. Is that the expression you usually had? What does the expression on your face tell you about the way you felt about yourself?

Look at your body. Is that the way you normally carried yourself? What does your posture tell you about your overall mood in that period of your life?

How do you think your relationships with friends and family were affected by your silence about your sexuality?

The Importance of the Gay Community

The gay community was a refuge from discrimination and abuse. Finding gay bars, groups, organizations, and other activities helped you develop a positive self-image and manage the stigma of being gay. When Hector discovered a gay cruising area in his neighborhood, he knew "this is where I belong." Later in life Ronald grew to accept himself through being around other gay men:

Being around gay men who are successful gay men, who are out and have been for years, it has somewhat blunted my fear of being discovered.

FAST FACT

Gay men who are involved in the gay community demonstrate

- greater acceptance of their sexuality
- better adaptation to aging

than gay men with little or no support in the community.[1]

As you review your history, you may find that the gay community played an important role in your process of self-acceptance. And you may be surprised to recognize that places such as cruising areas and bars were once as integral a part of building self-esteem as social clubs or organizations. Reflecting on your past will help you evaluate your current involvement in the gay community.

REFLECTION

What was it like when you were among others in the gay community? Look at a photo (or take a mental picture) of yourself among other gay people.

What changes did you see in your face and body from the earlier "photo"?

How do you think you physically changed as you moved between the gay and straight worlds?

Being Gay (HIV Positive and Older) Today

Changes in culture, economics, and acceptance of homosexuality have affected the gay community. Once you went to the Castro or

Greenwich Village to find gay men. Today, there are gay neighbor-hoods throughout the nation. And many gay men feel comfortable living in the cities, suburbs, and rural areas of this country outside of gay enclaves. But the breakdown of the "gay ghetto" has had other effects as well, as George recalls:

> **I look around the dog run and there's hardly any gay people there. So it's just a little strange for me. And I've been spoiled all my life living in a ghetto and enjoying feeling normal and now I don't feel quite so normal.**

George remembers walking out the front door of his West Village apartment house and being surrounded by other gay men. But now his neighborhood has changed, and he rarely sees gay men his age on the street. This change leaves George feeling "out of it."

The interests, activities, and language that make up gay identity continue to evolve. Terms such as "Friends of Dorothy" and refer-ences to Bette Davis are becoming less popular, as the need for coded language referring to homosexuality becomes less necessary and gay culture overlaps more with changing popular culture. Arthur feels like the gay community has lost cohesiveness and camaraderie:

> **Well, you don't have the orgies that there used to be. There is no longer the baths. There is no longer ... that whole life-style. There is no longer the theater life that then existed. There is no longer the ... gay element of having, if we may use it ever so [laughs] quote unquote, soirées in people's home, that is ... almost a dinosaur. That happens if you're lucky, once a year, where that used to be the norm. So you see all of these things have eroded.**

The community has become more diverse, and has greater inclusion of gay men, lesbians, bisexuals, and transgendered people of differing backgrounds. This progress may leave you feeling that you are no longer reflected in the community. Change can be uncomfortable. Rather than give in to that discomfort and lose a significant form of support, confront your prejudices. We all have them.

Age and HIV have changed you, too, and your interests may no longer reflect those of the gay community. Mario, for example, no longer feels as if he's a part of the gay community. He has little interest in bars, clubs, and the gay scene of his youth, and jokingly wonders if he is "no longer gay." Recognizing that you've changed over the years allows you to change your relationship to the gay community. Perhaps the "hang-outs" you had 20 years ago, if they still exist, no longer interest you.

REFLECTION

Take out those "photos" of yourself when you were in the closet and when you were with other gay people.
Now, look at your current facial expression and posture. Which of those two photos do you most closely resemble today?

The "Isms"

Just because attitudes toward gay people have improved in society does not mean that homophobia is a thing of the past. Homophobia has many forms of expression, including physical assault, threats of violence, and derogatory language. Discriminatory behaviors and policies continue to exist within organizations throughout this country, and in many places this kind of discrimination is still legal. For example, there is no federal law that expressly forbids workplace discrimination against lesbian, gay, bisexual, and transgender people. Less than half of all states specifically ban workplace discrimination in the private sector based on sexual orientation.[2] More subtle forms of discrimination, ones that make you feel uncomfortable and unwelcome, may be harder to identify, but they are still real and can affect your sense of safety and self-esteem.

FAST FACT

In a study of the lifetime victimization based on sexual orientation of 416 lesbian, gay, and bisexual adults aged 60 to 91 years, 75% (3/4) of the respondents reported some kind of sexual orientation victimization.[3]

Prejudice exists within the gay community as well. Experiences of ageism leave many men aging with HIV feeling ostracized from the community that they helped develop. At 56, Mark feels invisible in the gay community, noting, "Gay men, it's all about young, pretty boys, blah blah blah, whatever." Mario has gradually divorced himself from the "youth-oriented" culture of the gay community. And Peter described feeling "uncomfortable" and "misplaced" at a gay organization where he felt as if he was the oldest person in the room. Discrimination against middle-aged and older men within the gay community can be overt through exclusive policies or hostile remarks or can be more subtle expressions that make you feel unattractive, unworthy, and unwelcome.

AIDS stigma, too, can be common within the gay community. AIDS-related stigma is a significant feature of aging with HIV/AIDS that impacts mental health, coping, and social involvement.[4] The effects of AIDS stigma and the other "isms" as well as strategies to respond to discrimination will be discussed in more depth as we review the steps to optimal aging in Section III.

Joe recalls the time when his HIV support group decided to move rooms:

> In order to get to the group room we had to walk past the drop-in center. One time I heard this guy saying, "Those are the guys with AIDS." Other people had similar experiences, and some guys refused to join the group because they didn't want to have to deal with it.

Ron was active in an organization for gay African American men. During a meeting he heard two men gossiping about an HIV-positive member. Afraid that his status would be the subject of gossip, he stopped participating in the organization.

Experiences of prejudice and anticipating ageism and AIDS stigma can affect your interest in staying involved in the gay community, which once was so important to you. The gay community, however, can play an integral role in healthy aging. In Section III we will discuss strategies for addressing prejudice within the gay community.

RESEARCH REVIEW

Racism is a problem in the gay community, just as much as in the rest of society. A study of people living with HIV over 50 found that the "convergent disadvantages of race and age" manifest themselves in increased rates of infection, decreased health, rapid mortality, and lack of social supports among minorities,[5] as well as significantly more stressors compared with white people living with HIV over 50.[6]

To combat the effects of racism it's helpful to seek out the support of people who "get it."

Internalized homophobia is another significant "ism" that needs to be addressed when exploring changes in the gay community. Even if homophobic attitudes and discrimination might be less prevalent than in your youth, you were exposed to homophobia at a very young age. Before you knew you were gay you heard words like "faggot" or "queer." Perhaps you were present when the adults made a derogatory comment or you witnessed someone being teased or assaulted. These images get in there and affect the way we think about ourselves. Joe, for example, believes he is a very private person. He has never wanted his family to learn about his sexuality and for that reason has shied away from family gatherings. When he recently attended an event he realized that they didn't seem to care as much as he did and realized that he had been carrying a lot of shame that was affecting the way he interacts with others.

We must confront our internalized homophobia in order to adjust to change in the gay community and society as a whole, as Peter explains:

> **One salient point that I've learned is that I must fight off those internalizations. I must keep who I am here, free from those internalizations somehow. Because that's who I really am. And that's a challenge for me.**

> *Early in my career I was invited to co-lead a therapy group for men and women. Although I had a good deal of experience running groups*

*in the gay community, I had never facilitated a group that was pre-
dominantly straight. In the group I was nervous about my sexuality
being disclosed, and I avoided any references to people or places that
might have revealed that I was gay. I told myself that this was my
psychoanalytic stance and that I should be a "blank slate." But, in
truth, I was trying to hide my internalized homophobia.*

*Finally, a gay group member "outed" me. While it created a few
uncomfortable sessions, the group quickly moved on from the subject.
No one really cared about my sexual orientation.*

*Afterward I was more relaxed in the group. I became a more effec-
tive group leader when I was no longer carrying around a secret. My
need to hide my sexuality had more to do with my past shame than
anything that was going on in the group. Until I was forced to face the
issue, my unexamined internalized homophobia was negatively affecting me and my work.*

The gay community was once a significant source of support, as
you grappled with your identity, confronted homophobia, and
faced the challenge of HIV. Today, changes in the community and
in you may have left you less involved.

Reflect on how that shift in involvement has affected your emotional, social, political, and sexual well-being. Consider how you
can fill that gap today.

■ ASSIGNMENT ■

Fantasize about the perfect gay space for you. Maybe it would
be a monthly meeting for former hippies to talk politics and
hook up for sex. Or an opera group that meets weekly and
goes to performances. It's your fantasy—go for it. What part
of town would it be in? Would it be in a bar, center, or house?
Who would be there? What would you do?

Does anything like that exist? What would it take to create
such a group? Contact a friend who you think might be interested in joining.

You have reviewed how your gay identity has evolved over the
years—that changes in society, the gay community, and in your

interests have reshaped what being gay means to you in midlife and beyond. You've recognized how stigma has played a role in that evolution and how you must continue to face vestiges of that oppression that remain as expressions of internalized homophobia. In the next chapter we will talk about sex and how aging with HIV has impacted your sexual expression.

5

Let's Talk About Sex

You've lived through the gay sexual revolution, and if you weren't "doing it" all the time, most of your friends were. They were doing it everywhere they could—hook-ups, back room bars, parks, the baths. As Luis recalls:

> I was very promiscuous 'cause when I was young I was a very funtacious, very good looking young boy. I still consider myself good looking. I had a lot of sex. I went to a lot of continental baths. I went to a lot of orgies. I ... Fire Island, parks, you know [*laughs*]. I've done a lot.

Maybe you came out late, maybe you weren't a part of "the scene," or maybe you were in a monogamous relationship. The sexual revolution, and the sex scene of the 1970s and 1980s, still impacted your life.

A great deal has changed since then. AIDS and aging have reshaped your attitude about sex. Aging with HIV means finding a new path for yourself when it comes to sex. This chapter will help you review your sexual history and determine what is right for you today.

Sexual History

> Mark: I'm part of that generation where in the 70s everybody was doing it with everybody.

As Mark points out, for gay men of a particular generation, having sex, and lots of it, was the norm. George recalls spending most of his time in the pursuit of sex. And Mario remembers when sex was the "top priority."

Sex wasn't all just fun and games. Gay men were breaking the shackles of homophobia and rejecting the sexual norms of a society that oppressed them. Patrick explains how his sex life was a form of rebellion:

> Part of my sex life has been riddled with the homophobia of growing up the way I did and everything in a conservative, small, in the 50s and 60s ... place that in the 70s I did furtive, sexual things like go to bookstores and have sex. Have sex in Central Park. Have sex in men's rooms. Things that were trashy, were trashy. But ... I think that there's a part of me that needed to do trashy things to you know ... maybe I was expressing anger. I'm not sure.

The onset of the AIDS epidemic in the gay community stigmatized the sexual mores of the 1970s and 80s. Gay men developed shame and guilt about their sex lives. These feelings can make it difficult to look back on your sex life and to acknowledge the significant, often primary, role it played in your life. However, an inability to review your experience honestly can handicap you as you integrate sex into your life as a healthy element today.

REFLECTION

Can you list all your sexual partners and where you had sex with them? If not, can you come up with approximations for different periods of your life?

As you review your list consider the following:
How important was sex to you when you were younger?
How much time did you spend in the pursuit of sex?
Are there changes in your sex life throughout your life (frequency, partners, locations)?
What did you gain or lose from those experiences?
How do you feel when you look at that list?

Recognizing the important role sex once had in your life and how it has changed over the years helps you to evaluate your satisfaction with your sex life today.

Sex in Midlife

The gay sex scene has changed, and so have you. Shifts in libido, attitude, and opportunity have reshaped your sex life. Whether you are single or in a relationship, sex is a significant way in which you care for yourself and your partner. As you review how your sex life has changed, consider how actively you have participated in that shift.

Changes in Libido

Sometimes men at midlife feel as if their interest in sex has diminished. George doesn't have an appetite for sex, and is glad to see it go. He feels that sex once ruled his life, and appreciates the time he has to pursue other interests. Joe, too, believes that aging has reduced his sex drive:

> There's a natural dropping off point with sex too. I mean, I don't know if it's natural but it seems to be with … with the aging is that you don't … you know, you're not as sexually active as you once were.

After years of taking protease inhibitors Patrick developed diabetes and neuropathy, which eventually led to impotence. He tried taking oral medications to treat the impotence, but they stopped working. Now he uses injections directly into his penis. He said that at first it was difficult to inject himself. Now he's gotten used to it, and when the "opportunity arises," he's glad to have this option. He's also considering an implant, because despite the physical challenge he still wants to maintain an active sex life.

Jamie doesn't feel attractive anymore, and doesn't go out to pursue sex. But he adds with a smile: "But," he adds with a smile, "if a man falls in my lap…."

RESEARCH REVIEW

Some shift in sexual activity quantity and quality is common among men as they age. And research on men at midlife has demonstrated that although there are some changes in physiology that may affect sexual libido and change performance patterns, none of these changes is sufficient in the majority of men to significantly alter the interest and pleasure in a sensual and sexual life.[1]

For gay men at age 55, changes can become evident in erection, ejaculation, and anal pleasure[2]:

- Half of men have some erectile dysfunction, as well as changes in the position of their erection
- The size of the ejaculation shrinks and the time between orgasms increases
- Prostate enlargement occurs, which can affect anal pleasure

For men living with HIV, the physiological effects of aging on sexual function and libido can be complicated by the impact of HIV and HIV medications.

The brain is the most important organ when it comes to sex. If you're not into it, anxious about your performance, or afraid of infecting someone, those feelings can impact your ability to have and maintain an erection. Talk to your doctor if you are having sexual dysfunction to determine whether it is physiological, medication related, or emotional in order to determine the right course of treatment.

Changes in Attitude

Even if the drive is still there, aging with HIV creates a shift in your attitude about sex. Mark has much less interest in picking up men. While he used to meet men in bars, clubs, or on the street, now he occasionally meets men online, fools around with guys at the gym, or has sex with "play buddies" who he has known for years. He says that he doesn't feel like putting in the same effort anymore. Similarly, Luis feels like his priorities have shifted:

> I just don't want to get down and just have sex. I want to get down cause there's a feeling involved. There's a little connection of some sort. It's either I like your personality, I like your body, I like your face, I like you or ... but before it was just sex. That's it. You know? Put up or, sex! You know, and now it's not that. Now it's more that it's gotta be a connection. It's gotta be something that we can hook on. Something that we click ... it's just not sex. That's over.

And the presence of HIV shapes your sex life, as well. Luis is adamant about safer sex, even if it reduces the number of partners he can have. Mario, though, doesn't pursue sex at all. He is bored by safer sex and has lost his interest in sex:

> It's very safe. But that's boring too. It's kind of vanilla, you know, not to you know, get ... not to do it and ... and partake ... you know, with full enthusiasm.

The men talk about how aging with HIV has made them feel less attractive and diminished their interest in pursuing sex. Joe describes it this way:

> Another thing, too, is the image. Lipoatrophy, you don't feel attractive, so you don't even make an effort. You know, go there, period, because you don't want to be hurt and disappointed and rejected. Uh, which, you know, happens to all of us. Eventually, you know, it gets to a point, where it discourages us from pursuing that kind of lifestyle anymore.

Ronald believes the challenges of disclosure and fear of reinfecting himself and others are too much. He was diagnosed in 1990 and stopped having sex. He had a brief affair in 1999 and has been celibate ever since:

> So, that has a lot of, you know, restraints that it puts on you also because of communicable diseases, STDs. You don't know you can give and you can get. We can't afford to get much more, most of us.

Joe does not have sex with other people, but has a strong libido. He views masturbation as a way of taking care of himself, like healthy eating or working out. He has an active fantasy life, has sex toys, and has a collection of photos and stories on which to draw.

FAST FACT

In one study on HIV over 50, half of the respondents reported living a celibate lifestyle. The most common reason given for abstinence in this group was fear of infecting others.[3]

Tim, like several of the men I interviewed, continues to have an active sex life. Recently, he has been struggling with healthy sexuality. He feels that unsafe sex has become a problem. He feels compelled to have unprotected sex, but afterward feels guilt and shame. He worries about infecting others and exposing himself to diseases, and believes the pattern is hurting his self-esteem. Even so, he cannot stop. He calls it a "throwback to the good old days." Unsafe sex, as Tim explains, can be a denial of aging or a return to the past. It is also a dangerous behavior, even when you think the other person is HIV positive, that physically and emotionally damages you and your partner.

Sex within an intimate relationship also changes as we age. Arthur says that he and his partner have gone through many different periods. When they first got together it was "hot and heavy." After a while their sex life diminished and they each had more sex outside the relationship. Lately, he's been noticing less of an interest in having sex with other men and that the two of them are having sex more often. He finds the quality of the sex has changed too, and that it's "closer, more intimate."

Changes in Opportunity

Andy doesn't feel as though he has changed at all. He is still as interested in sex as he was as a young man. But he found that as he got older there were no longer places for him to go for sex. Many of the gay venues he frequented have been closed. Public spaces that he once cruised are now filled with young families. And the gay sex clubs available to him are expensive or filled with younger guys who reject him. For years, Andy felt his sex life was diminishing and he became depressed. Recently, he has reinvented himself as an S&M activist. He advertises on the web and now has men come to his apartment regularly.

Peter, however, is reluctant to meet men over the Internet. He is concerned about his safety and has heard that older guys can get robbed and victimized if they are not careful. The Internet has replaced bars and bathhouses as the place for fast and easy sex. There are websites out there for every taste and interest. Although ageism is still present on the web, there are also sites that cater to older men and the men who love them. But, as Peter points out, safety can be a real concern when you invite a stranger to your home or go to someone else's home. Only you can determine what level of risk is right for you, but when in doubt one rule of thumb that always works is to talk it out with someone else. You may feel hesitant about discussing your sex life with others, but chances are your friends may share some of the same concerns and can help you determine if you are taking unnecessary risks.

Many men turn to hustlers for sex. On the one hand, you can get what you want, when you want it. On the other hand, you will be spending money on a potentially illegal and unsafe encounter. Sometimes men find that they have spent much more time and money than they would have liked and finish feeling sexually satisfied, but emotionally empty.

REFLECTION

If you believe that sex could be negatively affecting your self-esteem, hurting your relationships with your partner, friends, or family, putting your job at risk, and getting you into legal or financial trouble, or if you believe that you are placing yourself in physical danger, then seek counseling. The Sexual Compulsives Anonymous website at www.sca-recovery.org has a list of 20 questions to determine whether their program is right for you. They help people develop their own sexual recovery plan, and to define sexual sobriety for themselves. Their literature states, "We are not here to repress our God-given sexuality, but to learn how to express it in ways that will not make unreasonable demands on our time and energy; place us in legal jeopardy; or endanger our mental, physical, or spiritual health."[4]

As a young man I considered sex to be a competitive sport in which strength, endurance, and agility received high marks. As I've gotten older, I've grown to appreciate the value of compassion, creativity, and patience in sexual expression.

■ ASSIGNMENT ■

Patrick Carnes, a leader in the field of sexual recovery, has conducted a great deal of research on healthy sexuality. The following assignment draws from his work[5]:

Review your sexual history. Describe at least eight events that were sexually/sensually positive for you. Determine what conditions made it special (what, where, and who you were with). Then, list five things these events all had in common. Finally, list five practical steps you can take to enhance your lovemaking.

1. Describe the sexual event. Example: A night on the beach with your first lover.
2. What made it special? Example: Ocean, stars, nature, time, hours of touching.
3. Commonalities. Example: Lots of touching, etc.
4. Steps: Set up some touch sessions with my partner. Talk about touching in my relationship. Make hugs a daily goal.

Sex was once an integral part of your identity and an important part of your social life in the gay community. As you've aged with HIV, physical changes, as well as shifts in attitude and opportunity, have reshaped your sex life. Sexual expression continues to be an important aspect of self-care as we age. This chapter has helped you to take some time to consider how satisfied you are with your sex life today. In the next chapter you will assess how aging with HIV has affected your intimate relationships.

6

Love and Marriage

An integral step toward successful aging, according to developmental theories,[1] involves the ability to form and maintain intimate relationships in early adulthood. Yet for gay men aging with HIV there have been a number of obstacles to developing an intimate relationship, including social pressures, internal struggles, lack of support for gay relationships (the "isms"), and the overwhelming disruption of AIDS in the gay community. Today, you may believe that aging and HIV have reduced your chances at finding love and that, as George says, "It's not in the cards."

However, intimate relationships come in many forms. Whether you are in a long-term relationship, are dating, have companionship with close friends, or have a pet, you can evaluate your satisfaction with these relationships and determine whether and how you can develop greater intimacy in your life.

The world is changing. Gay marriage, once a fantasy in the United States, is becoming a possibility in many states. To keep up with those changes, you must be able to reassess your ideas about intimacy at this stage of your life. This chapter will help you review your relationship history, consider dating and the obstacles to finding true love, and deepen your existing relationships.

Your Relationship History

Your relationship history affects your attitudes about intimacy today.

Mark lost "the love of my life" to AIDS. Mark and Dave met and fell in love when they were in their thirties. They had an active social life, bought a house in the country, and anticipated growing old together. Mark never had rose-colored glasses on. They had their arguments, had to work on keeping their sex life hot, and took each other for granted some of the time. They were both diagnosed with AIDS in the early 1990s, but while Mark responded well to treatments, Dave's health declined. Mark spent two years caring for his partner before he passed away.

After Dave's death, Mark never imagined entering another intimate relationship. He felt too much grief. He didn't think he had the capacity to love someone else. And he didn't want to risk going through that kind of loss again. Now he appreciates how much he gained from that relationship and wants something like that again. He feels enough time has passed to consider dating:

> I really and truly want to settle down. I would love to have someone to share something with. I would love to build a new chapter in my life.

As we age the ability to mourn becomes increasingly important, and memories of lost loves can give us strength and support. "One task of living out the last half of life is excavating and recovering all of those whom we loved in the first half," writes psychiatrist Dr. Vaillant.[2]

Joe and Mario did not lose their lovers to AIDS, but still feel "burned" by their experiences. They are reluctant to enter a relationship today.

Joe had a lover when he was in his forties. When it didn't work out, he was crushed and gave up on entering into another relationship. He felt that the hurt and loss were too much for him to risk:

> So that was two relationships that came to, like, unpleasant ends for me. And after that I just shied away from any kind of relationship and I got very casual about sex, the whole thing. That's all I had. Casual sex.

Mario had a long-term relationship with a man who was an alcoholic. He explains how he became an enabler in that relationship and that he watched his partner destroy everything in life—his friendships and his work—before he chose to leave the relationship.

He is concerned that if he gets into another relationship, he will fall into that same role again. Since then, he declares:

> I'm not even looking. I really have sort of stepped back from the whole thing. I'm very fatalistic about it.

Mark, Joe, and Mario give testament to the power the past can have over our lives in the present. Working through the grief, loss, and pain of past relationships helps us appreciate the good of those relationships, grow from those experiences, and be open to all that life has to offer in the present.

Our view of ourselves from the past also shapes our willingness to enter relationships in the present. Perhaps, like Andy, you never saw yourself as "a relationship-type person." Or, like George remembers, relationships were not "the thing" when you were younger. Peter felt that he was always too afraid of intimacy when he was a young man. When an opportunity arose in his forties, he had "a meltdown":

> And that hadn't happened in a long time. That's one of the areas of my life that I don't think I invite in often or even … I don't think I deal with myself on that level.

Peter says that his feelings of low self-esteem and shame were so strong that he never thought he could enter into a relationship. His "meltdown," as he calls it, led him into therapy, where he has worked through a great deal of internalized homophobia and is beginning to appreciate what he has to offer.

Tim, too, realizes that he has always had a wall up when it came to relationships:

> I think I always tried to maintain, and I think I was very successful because I was able to snow job everybody that ever entered my private area … for years. Probably over 10, no one, I mean a trick maybe came here but that, you know … we went to the bedroom, fucked and he left, sort of a thing. Or he spent the night, I made him breakfast and shoved him out the door. But there were no … there was no social … there was no chemistry here. There was no life here. There was no life here.

REFLECTION

Take some time to reflect on your past experience with intimacy.

Were you satisfied in those relationships?

Did you play a repeated "role" in your intimate relationships?

Were you burned by loss or rejection?

Can you remember the good parts of those relationships?

How do you think your experiences shape your willingness to enter a relationship today?

Dating

Perhaps, like George, you're getting ready to put yourself "on the market." Or you may have been dating for some time. You know the ups and downs of meeting men in the hopes of finding a relationship. Dating is a tool you can use to get to know someone else and yourself. Yet it also opens us up to fantasies, fears, and self-doubt. Understanding the obstacles (both anticipated and real) of dating when aging with HIV will help you be present with your experience.

One of the primary obstacles for anyone in the dating scene is confronting the fear of rejection. For gay men aging with HIV that fear is manifest in the disclosure of their HIV status and concerns about being "too old." Mark is concerned about meeting someone in a bar or a social situation and developing intimacy, only to be rejected when his HIV status is revealed:

> **I'm just thinking if I go out and I meet someone and they might be interested in me, that they may not necessarily want to follow through if they found out I happen to be HIV positive.**

Many gay men wonder about the right time to tell a potential partner about their HIV status. Disclosure is a frequently discussed topic in the support groups I run. Some men solve the "coming out" issue by meeting men only in HIV-positive groups, websites, social organizations, or positive dating events. Others make a point of telling potential partners their HIV status before or during their first encounter. Although these solutions do work, life does not always cooperate with our plans and, inevitably, if you are dating you will have to face the issue of disclosure. Just remember that anxiety about disclosure is normal, and that as long as you are okay with yourself, someone else's problem with your HIV status is exactly that—their problem.

Patrick is concerned that he is "too old" to reenter the dating world and that maybe that energy should be devoted to his career:

> **I mean aging and romance are not good partners, you know? It's hard at this age of 55 to be looking for a relationship, you know? And sometimes I worry about maybe it's easier, as hard as it is to get your doctorate, that it's easier to get your doctorate than it is to find a relationship.**

Mark feels that he is set in his ways and doubts whether someone would want him with all his "baggage." And George wonders how gay men of his age group meet:

> **Finding a relationship in a bar, it never worked before, why is it going to work now that I'm in my sixties?**

Where you go to meet someone depends on who you are looking for. Andy meets many younger gay men out there looking for "a daddy" online, but he doesn't want a relationship. Twenty years ago all George had to do was walk out the door of his West Village apartment if he wanted to meet a man, but now he has to cast a wider net.

First, ask yourself what qualities you want in a man. Do you have those qualities? Then consider what interests you and do more of that. Other suggestions for meeting men that came from the guys I interviewed include gay organizations, HIV-positive groups, mixers for older gay men, the opera, outdoors clubs, bars, friends of friends, and online dating sites.

Rather than act on your fears, consider what is getting in the way of your putting yourself out there. If you have an accurate assessment of yourself, and know your strengths and weaknesses, you are in a good position to meet someone real. Recognize how you've changed over the years. Consider where internalized homophobia, AIDS stigma, or ageism might be fueling fears of rejection. Just as you take an old pair of jeans out of the closet to see if they fit again, assess whether now is the time to start dating.

REFLECTION

When was the last time you went out on a date?
What have you done to put yourself out there?
What obstacles (fears) stand in your way?
List 10 things you can do to be more active in your pursuit.
Give yourself a deadline to accomplish each of those activities.

Relationships Today

FAST FACT

Being in a committed relationship has been demonstrated to have several beneficial effects for gay men,[3] including:

- A greater ability to manage depression and anxiety
- Assistance with health-related challenges
- An improved adaptation to aging

You have not been the only one to change. So has your partner. HIV, aging, changes at work, in the family, and in the community have affected him as much as you. Relationships need to grow to keep up with individuals in them. Now may be a time to reconnect with your partner and to reevaluate the strength and flexibility of your relationship.

Luis has been involved with a heterosexually married man for 20 years. Recently, he began feeling that he has not been getting enough from his partner, and began dating someone else. But he ended it with his new boyfriend and talked to his lover about his unmet needs. He knows that Manuel will always be his primary relationship:

> There's too much … there's memories, there's love, there's friendship, there's family involved—I'm the godfather to his daughter. It's just too much at stake. No one will ever take his place. I think I'll die with Manuel. In this type of relationship a lot of people don't understand.

Arthur always valued the independent nature of his relationship. He and his partner live separately and have an open relationship. He believes that this balance of freedom and care has encouraged him in his career and other areas of his life. Recently, when his health changed, he found that his lover's support became even more important. He has been glad to have his lover around more often.

RESEARCH REVIEW

Older adults report that their romantic experiences improve with age.[4] Factors that could contribute to successful relationships among middle-aged and older adults are:

- The accumulation of shared experiences
- Individual maturation
- And the support of others (children, family, community)

"Long-term relationships may be love's training ground—the settings where we master the skills required for emotional regulation, communication, and other relationship tasks," writes psychiatrist Dr. Vaillant.[5]

Relationships between two men have not been sanctioned by society, and the oppression gay men have faced has been an impediment to developing long-lasting relationships. Yet many couples have bonded, and flourished, despite societal discrimination. And sometimes gay couples have unified against the front of the homophobic pressure from the outside world. Gay men have created their own definition of healthy relationships, and gay couples follow many different models. What is most important is that the relationship work for both of the members involved. Successful relationships involve constant "fine tuning" to respond to each individual's changing needs. One tool for enhancing communication and keeping the spark alive in relationships is instituting "date night," where you and your partner get out of the day-to-day routine and go on a date. Figure out what you need to do refresh your relationship.

REFLECTION

How has your relationship changed over the years?
What brought you together with your partner?
What do you get out of your relationship today?
How could your relationship improve? What do the two of you do to work on your relationship?

When I was in my twenties I rejected the idea of gay marriage. I believed that anything that smacked of conforming to a heterosexual normative status was wrong for the gay rights movement.

At age 42 I married my partner of 8 years in California and threw a party in New York for all our friends and family. The marriage created unexpected changes in our relationship and the security we each felt as a result of the commitment has deepened our emotional and sexual connection in subtle ways. I am able to appreciate why I was against gay marriage in the past and see how time and experience have altered my perspective.

Gay men aging with HIV at midlife have developed many creative approaches to having much-needed intimacy. After their relationship ended Hector and his ex-boyfriend continued to live together. At first, the arrangement was purely financial, but now he finds he relies on his ex-partner for emotional support as well. Mario has a group of really close friends. They get together regularly, go to museums and the opera together, take each other to doctor appointments, and check in on each other with regular phone calls. Jamie lives for his dog. He never lets himself get too depressed and makes sure to take care of his physical health, because he knows he has to be there for his beloved pet.

Review your satisfaction with the intimacy in your life.

■ **ASSIGNMENT** ■

Draw a large circle and place yourself in the center. In the circle write the names of your most intimate relationships.

Consider why you call them "intimate?"

What do you share with each? Are there things you keep from some of them?

Are there circles of intimacy within that circle?

Write down one piece of information you could share with each person (a secret, a story from your past). Write a feeling you could let the person know (how you care about them, a wound, an apology). Write one intimate act (a visit, gift, hug) that you could do to deepen that relationship.

Now, choose one thing to do right now. Consider doing this on a regular basis.

Who else would like to be included in that circle if given the chance?

Aging with HIV involves reevaluating your ideas about intimate relationships at this point in your life. In this chapter you have reviewed your relationship history and considered how it has affected your attitudes today. You've viewed your interest in and obstacles to dating. And you have assessed your satisfaction with the intimacy in your life. The only question now is to determine whether you want greater intimacy in your life, and to ask yourself how you are going to get it. In the next chapter you will reconsider your changing role in the family.

7

In the Family

Just as a child's development into adolescence creates shifts to which both the child and family must adapt, entering midlife involves creating a new role. Caring for aging parents or young children, shifts in sibling dynamics, and the death of a parent mean new responsibilities and new relationships. Even if you have not followed a normative heterosexual family structure, the dynamics in your family have changed with aging, death, births, and development. This chapter will help you to review your history and reassess your current place in the family.

FAST FACT

Middle-agers are often referred to as the "sandwich generation," simultaneously caring for children and aging parents. This family role offers us a perspective on our development, allows us to consider new options beyond the self, and helps us recognize our own mortality.[1]

Family History

> Peter: Despite the differences that we have with our parents, because we all know our own identity ... we have differences and inevitably we're not too far from where we started.

Your ability to gain perspective on your family history, to recognize its influences, and to acknowledge your similarities and differences to family members gives you the freedom to choose what you want to carry from your past into midlife and beyond. Mark talks with pride about his father's accomplishments. He admires the fact that as a poor, recent immigrant his father was able to build a business and hold public office. He always felt loved and cared about by his father, and feels that his father's support was significant to his success in his career. Arthur feels that as an only child his parents gave him a great deal of attention. He believes that they instilled in him a sense of self-confidence and self-love. Joe grew up in a large family. When his parents immigrated to the United States he was left in the care of his grandparents for several years. He felt loved by his grandparents but wonders if that absence affected his self-esteem. Luis had an aggressive, alcoholic father who he avoided. He thinks that his anxiety with boys at school was a direct result of his experience with the only other male in the household, and that he has had difficulty relating to men in his adulthood as a result. Still, he was always close to his mother and sister and has developed close bonds with women throughout his life.

The influences of childhood are subtle and varied. Only you can determine the effect your family history has had on your identity and development and if today, as Peter points out, you are not too far from where you started.

RESEARCH REVIEW

Family life is the context in which children develop. These early relationships shape our identity and our relationships with others in the outside world in childhood[2] and in later life.[3]

In his book *Aging Well*, George Vaillant, M.D., gives us a unique perspective on family history and its influence in later life adjustment. The *Study of Adult Development* includes three long prospective studies following a total of 814 diverse groups of men and women continuously for six to eight decades. The research includes both subjective and objective reports of their physical and mental health. Vaillant's analysis offers insight into the influences on healthy aging.

Vaillant finds a complex relationship between childhood and old age. Contrasting the experience of those with the bleakest childhoods with that of the most "sunny" he finds that at midlife, childhood history had an effect on mental and physical health. For example, he found that at age 53, more than a third of the 23 men with bleak childhoods already suffered from chronic illnesses, whereas among the 23 men with the warmest childhoods, only two were chronically ill. However, he also found that by age 75 this correlation broke down and there was little relationship between the quality of childhood and objective physical health.[4]

Family history affects our physical and mental health in later life. However, aging offers us opportunities to build new identities, create new bonds, and develop in new ways that effectively "rewrite" the influences of history.

Family and Sexual Identity

One defining experience for gay men is the handling of sexual identity in the family. Experiences of estrangement, hiding, and acceptance can have lasting affects on your identity and development. Arthur believes that his parents' acceptance of his homosexuality gave him the confidence to succeed in his career. Patrick knows that having an aunt who was a lesbian significantly helped him accept his sexuality and develop self-esteem. As Jamie points out, his mother was a source of constant support for him:

A lot of people's parents push them away. It seemed mine got closer.

Estrangement from family can be acutely felt at midlife. Andy felt that his family was not going to accept his homosexuality. He moved away and had little contact with them. His mother's death came with an unexpected call from his sister. This call made him consider the impact their estrangement had on him and his relationship with his sister.

Luis hid his sexuality from his homophobic father. His father used to speak openly about his antigay attitudes. He bragged about having beaten up a guy in his youth for looking at him "the wrong way." When Luis shared the secret of his homosexuality with his mother, but refused to tell his father, this created even more distance between the two of them. Now, he sometimes looks in the mirror and sees his father looking back at him. It is a challenge for him to recognize that he shares traits with the father he worked so hard to get away from.

Joe always kept a distance from his family, and a recent family reunion was a source of much discomfort for him. Although he wanted to attend, he feared their reaction to his appearance. He believed that he had the look of AIDS, and that if his family saw him they would know the secret of his sexuality and diagnosis. Joe ultimately attended the reunion and was surprised by their acceptance. He cries when he remembers the warm greeting he received from his two grown nephews. He plans on staying connected with them and their families.

Examining the impact of your family history on your development and identity can be a lifelong process. Peter is in psychotherapy to make sure he doesn't get stuck repeating old family patterns. Families, just like individuals, have the potential for change, if given the opportunity. As you continue reading this chapter, consider whether you have gotten stuck in your family history and if you have allowed your relationships within the family and your family role to evolve over time.

■ ASSIGNMENT ■

A genogram is graphic depiction of relationships within a family. The following description on how to construct a genogram is adapted from the work of McGoldrick and Gerson[5]:

You are making a map with figures representing people and lines marking their connections to one another. The figures are either a box for a male or a circle for a female. Use double lines when you draw the box representing you.

There are different types of lines to depict connections. Two people who are married are connected by lines that go down and across (in heterosexual marriages the husband is on the left and the wife on the right). You can write *m.* with the date they were married above the horizontal line. If they were separated write *s.* plus the date or *d.* plus date for date of the divorce. You will also write one slash for separated and two for divorced across the line. For unmarried couples you use a dotted line and the date they met, started living together, or other commitment. Multiple marriages are difficult to depict.

With that introduction to the basics of genogram construction, begin making a genogram to represent your immediate family. Above you include your parents and above them your grandparents. Include your parents' marriages/divorces, siblings, and children. Next to you place your significant others (present and past). This level also includes your siblings. Below you place your children, if any. On the same level you would place your sibling's children, if they have any. Finally, draw a circle using a dotted line around those members of your family who live in the same household.

My simple genogram appears as shown in Figure 7.1.

RECORDING FAMILY INFORMATION

Add demographic information near each person's symbol. Age is included within the symbol; dates of birth above; and location, education, and occupation on the side of the symbol. You can include functional information, such as medical conditions, career success, emotional well-being, and behavioral attributes (such as excessive drinking or absenteeism from work). Critical family events including moves, job changes, or environmental traumas can be recorded on the page or in a separate chronology.

You can use different lines to symbolize the various types of relationships between two family members. Clinicians use the following terms to describe possible ways of relating: very close or "fused"—triple lines; poor or conflictual—jagged lines; close—double lines; estranged—broken line; distant—dotted line.

You can ask yourself the following questions: What was your relationship to each of your parents? Was your mother overprotective, critical? Were you her confidante? And your father—was he tough? Distant? Supportive?

Now, consider your parents' relationships with their parents and siblings. Can you see why they parented you the way they did?

Do you recognize any patterns in your relationships today that go back to your family? (Are you a caregiver, perfectionist, or martyr? Are you aloof, critical, or people pleasing?) How did you "learn" to be that way?

Aging Parents

As our parents age we gain perspective on their individuality and their frailty. Caring for aging parents can be difficult and time consuming, especially for adult children who have moved away and are involved in their own lives. However, the experience can be rewarding as well—helping adult children to recognize that they have something to offer their parents. The time spent gives parent and adult child the chance to resolve differences and heal old wounds. In midlife the death of a parent gives us a new role in the family. When we become one of the older generation, we can take on new responsibilities within our extended families.

Patrick finds it works the other way around. He relates his mother's ailments to his own history with AIDS. He can identify with her feelings and draws from his experience when he talks to her about living with illness, dependence, and mortality. Mario, though, keeps his illness from his older mother, saying, "why burden her now?" Tim is still adapting to having older parents.

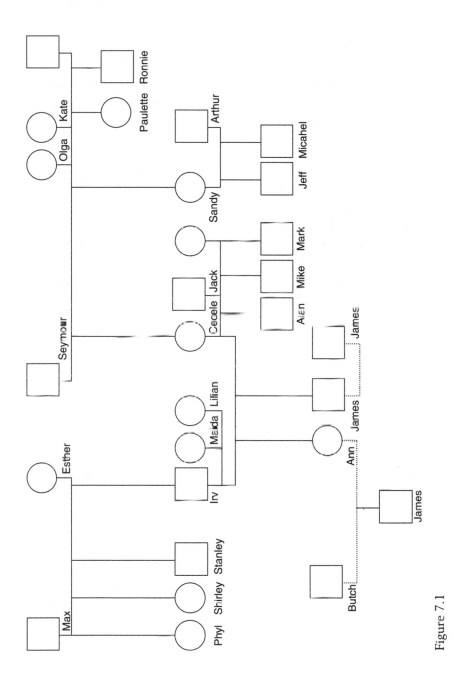

Figure 7.1

He never thought that he would live to experience their aging and the eventual role reversal involved in taking care of them.

Jamie believes that caring for his mother when she was ill changed his personality and view about life. He explains:

And then, like I said, as she got sicker I knew that my priorities had to change. That I had to stop thinking about me and think about her now.

Having faced your own mortality and experienced the loss of friends and lovers may alter your experience of a parent's death. However, it does not relieve you from the process of mourning. The death of Jamie's mother was difficult, but he feels that she is always with him. Hector believes that his mother's death triggered his drug use. Peter finds that his perspective has changed since the death of his parents. Grieving a parent's death includes mourning what you did and did not receive from them. The process of grieving a parent can be made more difficult when there is estrangement or unresolved tension between parent and surviving child.

REFLECTION

Reconsider your role in the family.

Go through the genogram and place an x through the symbol of everyone who is deceased and mark the date of death next to the birthday. Think about how your family handled their illness and death. Was there drama? Stoicism? Who cared for them? Was there conflict around a will? How involved were you?

Who cares for/cared for your parents? Consider whether your involvement in your parents' illness or death was influenced by your role in the family. How did your position in the family change? How has it changed you as a person?

Sibling Relationships

Your brothers and sisters have been aging and changing, too. Although Peter was never close to his parents, his brother was, and still is, his best friend. Mark's relationship with his family has changed over the years. After the death of his parents, he stays in touch with his siblings with occasional phone calls and visits. The belief that his family is there for him is more important than day-to-day involvement:

> They play a very big role. Are they a sort of support or guidance? Not really. I know they're there for me. And I know they love me dearly and I know that if I ever needed anything they would be there. They were there when I lost Gary. They were there when I lost my best friend Don. They were there when, you know, when I lost my other friends. So you know they've been around. They're kind of like your anchor.

REFLECTION

Once again, return to your genogram and consider your relationships with your siblings.

Which child were you—youngest, oldest, middle, only?

How did the kids get along? Were there alliances? Did they shift over time?

Do you see patterns in the way you related to your brothers and sisters in your relationships with friends? If you were an only child, how do you think that influences your friendships?

As you have gotten older, how have your relationships with your siblings changed? How have old patterns of relating continued?

Do these patterns impact your ability to make the most of those relationships today?

Children

Having children in your life gives you the opportunity to play, reexperience your own childhood, see what you have to offer, and consider the future. Joe had a son when he was in his teens. He does not know much about his son's life and is considering whether he should try to develop a closer relationship to him at this point in his life. Luis, too, has a child from an earlier relationship. He is very proud of his son and his achievements and enjoys hanging out with his now adult son. He feels as though his son keeps him young, and he is constantly learning from him.

FAST FACT

Unlike younger people with HIV/AIDS, middle-aged and older people living with the virus do not rely significantly on family for emotional or instrumental support.[6]

Tim feels that his relationship with his niece and nephew gives his life meaning. He invites them to stay with him in New York. He talks to them openly about sex, drinking, and HIV. He wants to offer them guidance and acceptance, two things he felt weren't there for him as a teen and young adult. George's good friend has two young children. He loves getting on the floor and playing with them.

REFLECTION

Return to your genogram. Does it include children? What is your relationship like with the children on the genogram? Would you like to deepen that connection? Would you like to add more young people to your genogram?

As a gay man at midlife you may have a complex relationship with your family. You may have been estranged from your family. You may have members of the family who have been of significant support. Perhaps you are caring for an aging parent or mourning their loss. Your life could include children. And you could have a "nonconventional" or "alternative" family consisting of partners, friends, siblings, nephews, nieces, and their children. Whatever your family constellation, relationships change, and aging with HIV involves adapting to the changing dynamics between you and your family members.

I recently celebrated my 42nd birthday with my family. At first, I was quite reluctant to do so. I had little interest in celebrating this birthday, and even less in giving up a Saturday, paying for a rental car, and schlepping out to Long Island.

But, after a few hours of eating, laughing, and having a generally good time, I surprised myself because I didn't want to leave. Looking around the room I realized that this was my family: my husband and dog; my aunt, who keeps us updated on the New York theater scene; my sister, who seems to take care of everything and everybody; my teenage nephew, who is in a band; and my parents, who, now that they have been divorced longer than they were married, get along great. And I love them all.

And that's when I recognized that I was middle-aged. Because not only had my birthday become an excuse to spend time with my family, but I preferred to be with them that day than partying with friends. My role in the family has shifted. I drove out to Long Island because my father can no longer make the drive himself. And to see the look on my nephew's face when I opened the Star Trek card he picked out for me.

I am taking my position in the middle of a multigenerational family. I hope I can make the most of this time, as long as it lasts. fast fact

Middle-agers are often referred to as the "sandwich generation," simultaneously caring for children and aging parents. This family role offers us a perspective on our development, allows us to consider new options beyond the self, and helps us recognize our own mortality.[1]

■ ASSIGNMENT ■

Return to your genogram and draw a circle around your name. In it include your "chosen family." My family tree includes my closest friends, their children, and my dog.

Now, look at your tree as a whole: What do you feel? Are you satisfied with your tree? Do you wish it was fuller?

What steps can you take to deepen the relationships with members of your family? What additions can be made to your chosen family?

You may need to step out of an old family role to create those improvements!

8

What About Work?

At the beginning of each interview I asked the participants to tell me about themselves. Most of the time, the men described themselves by their work, present or former. "I was an art teacher." "I'm a nurse." "I was working in import/export." They identified themselves by what they did for a living. But as the interviews progressed I realized that aging with HIV reshaped that relationship to work, and a far more complex picture arose. For many, what they did for a living became far less important. And, now, they were reconsidering what role work should play in their lives.

Our work is an important part of how we define ourselves and our relationship to the world. As Erikson explained, "Mature man needs to be needed."[1] Employment, either paid or voluntary, plays a significant role in our mental health at midlife. Yet many people living with HIV no longer work, and have difficulty imagining how the benefits of work could outnumber the challenges inherent in holding down a job while living with a chronic illness. In this chapter you will consider what productivity means as you age with HIV, and identify the benefits and challenges of being in "retirement."

Productivity at Midlife

Continued productivity is integral to healthy aging. Although the primary benefit of work is making money, there are other less tangible results. Being involved in either paid or unpaid employment provides structure, an opportunity for interaction with others, and a way to stay active and involved. Luis thinks that keeping busy relieves his stress, and that if he weren't working he would be "biting his nails." Peter states that the primary reason he works is that he needs the money. Yet he also feels that the active pursuit of work is motivating:

It's something very ... strong about not wanting to ... not wanting to what? Work keeps me going. The pursuit of it. Looking for it keeps me very active, I guess. Very involved. It's just very full and moving. I don't want anything that's sort of ... smacks of stopping. Of ... of easy. Of resigning. Of any kind of resignation in it.

RESEARCH REVIEW

Work and career play an integral role in development for men at midlife. The world of work has been described as a potent motivator in this period[2] and an arena to work out inner conflicts.[3] At midlife men either come to recognize that their dreams have not been realized, or consider the meaning and value of their success.[4] And career consolidation or transforming a job or hobby into a career has been viewed as an integral task in adult development.[5] For gay men the salience of work at midlife has been given even greater emphasis. It has been argued that childless gay men have fewer opportunities for generativity than heterosexual men at midlife and that they gain esteem through productivity in the workplace.[6] Discrimination against one's race, ethnic background, class, and sexual orientation, among others, can impact one's opportunities for education and career advancement. Gay men aging with HIV must be open to creating alternate paths toward identity development, social involvement, and life satisfaction at midlife.

There are many emotional benefits to work. Work can be a source of self-esteem and provide a sense of accomplishment. Mark feels a sense of camaraderie with his co-workers, many of whom are gay. As his health improved, Patrick decided to switch careers. Now he is in the health care industry and likes the fact that his work allows him to "give back." Arthur does not get paid while writing his book, but he still finds the work very satisfying. He is glad that he will be "leaving something behind."

Careers also offer leadership opportunities to guide the next generation. In the field of gerontology this process is often referred to as generativity. Generativity is an integral step in adult development in which we give of ourselves for the benefit of others, including acting as a consultant, guide, mentor, or coach.[7] Many of the men discuss participation in my study as a form of generativity— a way to give back to the community.

When my lover, Roger, died, I was 24 years old and working as a cocktail waiter. His illness and death reshaped my life. I developed a greater understanding of the meaning of life and became aware of a world beyond myself. I returned to school and became a social worker. I worked in the field of AIDS care for over two decades.

Now that I am in midlife I recognize that Roger and many other men like him never had the opportunity to grow into middle age and beyond. I carry Roger's memory on through my work. This book is dedicated to him. It is my opportunity to be generative in midlife.

Challenges

Although there are many benefits from work, caring for your health can be a full time job as well. Medical appointments, complex medication regimens, fluctuating health, fatigue, and illness can make maintaining employment seem impossible. George explains that although he wants to work, or even volunteer more, it is imperative for his health that he avoid stress:

> Now, I'm starting to think that maybe if I could find something that was maybe even two days a week, 'cause I have to be very careful about not getting.... Stress is the killer. Stress is what kills you. And I'd rather be poor than stressed.

The idea of returning to a career put aside because of illness, or of beginning a new one, can feel daunting. You may feel less competitive because you have spent years out of the workforce. Hector wants to return to work, but feels that no one will want him because of his age. Interviewing for paid and volunteer employment involves overcoming emotional obstacles. Sometimes Patrick wonders why he's working so hard at this point in his life:

> This is a crucial piece of this, that I am 55 and there are those things about 55 that make you want to say, oh just relax, you know? Just, I mean, life, what is it? If you live to be a hundred you got 45 more years, maybe you should just really enjoy yourself, you know? But on the other hand because that was snatched out of my life in my late 30s and throughout my 40s, I'm scrambling to have those experiences that I should have had when I was younger. You know, but since I didn't have them, so I'm conflicted between being 55 and going, well, gee you're 55, you know, it's hard to get out of bed, just relax! Enjoy your life, you know? Don't work so hard. And then this other part that's still hungry.

Employment offers the potential for financial, social, and emotional benefits. Yet HIV has dramatically impacted your involvement in work and your pursuit of a satisfying career. Reevaluating your relationship to work can help you consider what role work should play in your future.

REFLECTION

Evaluate your work (paid or unpaid) satisfaction.

Does your work life make you feel good about yourself and your abilities?

Do you have contact with others through your job?

Do you feel connected to something bigger than yourself?

Do you have opportunities to mentor younger or less experienced colleagues?

Does your job provide you with challenges?

Do you feel adequately compensated?

Are you actively pursuing a career change?

Retirement

For some, retirement at the end of a satisfying career is a rewarding period of self-generated productivity. But for many, retirement can be stressful, especially when it is unplanned, involuntary, or a result of health challenges, and leaves you unable to support yourself financially. For many of you, HIV came just as your career was taking off. You were forced to make decisions as to whether to prioritize your health care at the expense of your work and as to when you needed to cut back or leave work entirely. You must consider your experience of "retirement" and your feelings about being retired in order to make the most of this phase of your life.

FAST FACT

When circumstances beyond your control intervene and impact career development at midlife, the possibilities for depression and stagnation increase.[8]

Retirement is a challenging shift at any age, but when separation from work comes with health complications at midlife or younger, it can be traumatic. Mario remembers that the decision to quit work and take care of his health "was hell." He tried to balance his health and his job, while hiding his diagnosis, but eventually it got to be too difficult. George believes he could have kept working longer, but felt that he was forced out when his boss learned of his diagnosis. Patrick feels as if it was a choice to leave work when he no longer could physically manage the job. He still misses his old career in the theater, and wonders how far he would have gone if his health hadn't gotten in the way.

The trauma of forced retirement can leave scars on your psyche and may be impacting your attitude toward your life today. Patrick is very productive. In midlife he returned to school, got a graduate degree, and has developed a new career. Peter does "just about anything" to make money. His day is filled with work-related activities, including temp work, playing the piano professionally, and going to auditions. Yet he believes that at his age he should be "further along." Be careful to make sure that self-defeating atti-tudes and judgments about your career success don't hold you back from receiving satisfaction from your productivity today.

FAST FACT

Rewarding retirement involves:

- Replacing workmates with new friends and companions
- Rediscovering how to play (through sports, cards, or other competition)
- Finding creativity
- Building lifelong learning[9]

The challenge of retirement involves making the most of your time. Mark was offered a buy-out at his company. He wasn't quite sure what he would do with his time, but decided this was an opportunity to begin a "new chapter." He has since taken classes in real estate, immersed himself in yoga, and returned to painting. While sometimes he feels as if he's "all over the place," he also appreciates how retirement has given him an opportunity to redis-cover himself. The key to a satisfying retirement is to be intellectu-ally, creatively, and physically stimulated while remaining involved with other people.

■ ASSIGNMENT ■

Make a list with four columns and write at the top: "people," "play," "creativity," and "learning."
Now, fill in the columns with five replacements for your work life that you are (or could be) involved in.
Can you add five more in each column?

Your view of yourself has changed as you've been aging with HIV. Once you defined yourself by your career, but then HIV reshaped your priorities. Productivity is still an important aspect of your life. Reviewing your relationship to work allows you to decide whether your work life reflects your current interests and challenges. As you have reviewed the changes you have undergone both in work and retirement, I hope you have seen the connections between the two. The benefits and the challenges of both work and retirement are very similar. In each, you must feel productive, connected, generative, and creative in order to be satisfied. In the next chapter you will evaluate how you've changed internally as you've been aging with HIV.

9

My, How You've Grown

In the past eight chapters you've identified changes in the AIDS epidemic, your physical body, the gay community, your social circles, your sex life, your intimate relationships, your role in the family, and your work life. And as you've evaluated your adaptation you've begun to recognize how much you've changed in the process, as Luis has:

> Because I don't think of the virus has changed me. I think what's changed me is my age. My wisdom. My experiences. Times. I don't think it's been the virus. I don't think the virus has slowed me down. I think I've slowed down because I'm seeing life different. Because of being a middle-aged man. Not because I'm a gay man, or because I'm an HIV man. Because I'm a middle-aged man. And I see life and I see people and I see the times and I see how things have changed.

For some of you these internal shifts have gone unrecognized. Not until you are forced to stop and think about it do you realize how much your interests, priorities, and even identity have evolved. This chapter will explore your psychological, emotional, and spiritual growth.

RESEARCH REVIEW

The capacity for internal change is an integral aspect to healthy aging. In his analysis of the *Longitudinal Study of Adult Development*, Vaillant defines four personal qualities that serve as protective factors against the challenges of life and assist in healthy aging:

- Future orientation (the ability to anticipate, to plan, and to hope)
- The capacity for gratitude and forgiveness
- Empathy (the ability to see the world as it seems to others and to love)
- The desire to do things with people[1]

Our futures are not written in stone, but, rather, it is our ability to adapt to changes in our environment that offers us the greatest possibility of healthy aging.

Recognizing Middle Age

This section feels like the beginning of some Catskill comedian's stand-up routine: "You know you're middle-aged when ..." Aging is a constantly evolving process and the internal changes that have occurred as a result are not always evident. We often rely on "age-markers"—experiences that trigger the recognition of aging. As you read what the men have to say, consider what events trigger an awareness of aging in you.

Peter found that reaching a certain "number" made him recognize his aging:

> **Ever since I turned 50 ... it's sort of a ... not a resignation in a bad way but sort of an acceptance of being 50.**

Luis feels his aging when he experiences his physical limitations:

> **Oh, maybe when I feel a little sick or I feel a little tired. I say, damn, I'm tired. Well, I'm 51 years old. Shit, when I was young I could run the world and didn't get tired.**

George knows he's middle-aged when he considers how many people he has lost:

> Something popped through my head about getting old. Seeing so many ... I mean, I see many, many more young people than I see people my age around. Most of my friends are dead. I have ... very few friends that are left. But that makes me feel old. That all that is changing.

Hector has to reevaluate his aging when he looks in the mirror, even when friends say he looks the same:

> You know, OK, I'm getting older. [*laughs*] But ... but basically, if you see all my pictures through my age ... I got all those pictures, I look the same. You know, ... everybody says, oh my god you look the same!

Luis doesn't feel as though he's changed. But he is forced to recognize his aging when he gets treated like "an old guy":

> Forty and over. The old people. You make me look like a senior citizen already? So I took it like offensively but I just ... I'm a kid. But I don't know. I don't ... I don't know what 51 is supposed to feel like.

Joe didn't know he was changing until he looked at the people he was spending time with. When he realized that he had little in common with these younger friends, he sought out companionship with men closer to his own age:

> So I began to need people that were older to share with, because I no longer had that much in common with younger people in that sense. And I lacked the perspective of an older person. Or older peers and people, which led me to SAGE.

Arthur becomes aware of his aging when he tries to look for work. He sees his age in the way he gets treated by potential employers:

> I think that the only time it comes to play is when I realize that the job market is no longer there for me. That's when I become aware of it.

Tim finds that it's harder to see his aging because he doesn't have children. He feels that seeing a child's development would help him recognize his own:

> I think of middle aged as being almost a grandparent, which I am not and won't be, because I never had children. So I don't really have anything to look at to see, oh look she's graduating from high school, or he. Or my dog died and he was or she was 20. I don't have that stuff that I think other people and now I can't say heterosexuals, but other people have that. You know, their children are graduating from high school or college or getting married or …

Birthdays, physical health, loss, appearance, the perceptions of others, intergenerational attitudes, and experiences of discrimination are all age markers. They trigger in us an awareness of our own aging. These may be uncomfortable at times, but, as Tim points out, without these reminders we have no mirrors to see that we are changing. Recognizing that your identity has shifted as you've grown older is an important part of reevaluating your needs and desires at this life stage.

Psychological Development

In the field of gerontology there is some debate about whether we change at all as we age, or whether we just become more like who we already are. Do our identities evolve as we grow older? Do we continue to develop psychologically, emotionally, and spiritually in middle and older age? Do we mature, or just get more stuck in our ways?

For Mark, both arguments are true. On the one hand he has seen an increasing inflexibility in his attitude as he's gotten older:

> You know, you get to a certain cycle and habits and behaviors. I mean I certainly am aware of how I've gotten older in my likes, dislikes … things that I have no patience for that I used to have patience for.

Yet he is also open to change. In midlife he took an opportunity to retire from his job, not to sit around, but to begin a new chapter in his life:

It was, you know, it was the right thing to do to take advantage of … of a new chapter and write something different.

I find evidence of psychological development throughout these men's stories. However, sometimes it may be hard to determine whether this maturation is due to age or HIV, or a combination of the two, as Joe points out:

And it, from there on there was a double change that I had to go through. Not only the aging because … or the middle age business of going from the young person to a middle aged person, but also acquiring a whole new approach to life.

RESEARCH REVIEW

Life stage theorists believe that our psychological development continues throughout the lifespan. They conceptualize aging as a series of stages that follow each other in sequence. Each stage can be defined by a basic theme or conflict. As children we master the conflicts of "Basic Trust vs. Mistrust," "Autonomy vs. Shame," "Initiative vs. Guilt," and "Industry vs. Inferiority."

In adulthood we pass through four additional stages:

- "Identity vs. Identity Diffusion"—In adolescence and young adulthood, we develop a sense of ourselves separate from our family of origin.
- "Intimacy vs. Isolation"—In young adulthood we develop the capacity to form close bonds with others and enter into interdependent, reciprocal, and committed relationships.
- "Generativity vs. Stagnation,"—In midlife we can either be generative through procreation, production, and creativity, passing on our knowledge to others, or stagnate in self-absorption and shrink away from youth, productivity, and the concerns of others.
- "Integrity vs. Despair"—In older age we gain experience of a world order and spiritual sense. Accepting that our life has been as it should be helps us avoid fear of death, despair, and disgust.[2]

Life stage theory has been criticized for being too general and too idealist: that it does not give much indication of the ways in which cultural differences, sex differences, or social class differences interact with this general developmental progression[3] and that midlife gay men and lesbians "may be creating a unique developmental trail through the middle years of life."[4]

Given these caveats, the life stage model of adult development can be used as a road map for understanding where we might be and for mastering certain challenges in order to deal more effectively with the losses of aging, and continue to grow beyond ourselves in adulthood.

Reordered Priorities

One way to understand maturity is to see how your interests have changed with time. Or, as Mario puts it:

> It's about priorities shifting. Things that used to be important no longer are.

Patrick's midlife career change is an example of how aging with HIV reshaped his priorities. He describes his decision to do something more meaningful with his life in middle age:

> I just said goodbye to the previous life, to the previous definition of who I was. I wanted to do something more meaningful.

Luis believes that aging has matured him and that has affected how he treats himself and others:

> Yes, yes, definitely my priorities have changed. Oh yes. I take life more seriously. I don't engage in unsafe sex. I ... take care of myself. I watch my friends. I don't make friends like I used to. I have a lot of acquaintances and I got a few friends.... I matured in every way. A lot different. Age has a lot to do with it. Wisdom. I'm substituting the club, for the jobs. I'm substituting the drugs, for the volunteer. I'm substituting one thing for another, but this is more constructive, this is more

beneficial. When I see the effect on others, it's so rewarding. I've done something for someone. It's not all about me now.

Joe and Jamie point out that shifting priorities can sometimes leave one feeling out of it:

Joe: But the thing about that is, is that when you change and people still want you to be in that same role, that's a little disconcerting because ... you know, although I don't see that those ... I don't see those people anymore.

Jamie: My social life is very small. When I was younger, all I wanted to do is party, party, party, and now that I'm older things change. I don't feel the same. I prefer to stay home.

Shifting priorities from immediate concerns, short-term pleasures, or self-directed activities toward a broader outlook—thinking beyond yourself and being able to see a bigger picture—demonstrates psychological development with age.

RESEARCH REVIEW

People living with HIV over the age of 50 report that age offers some advantages:

- With age comes wisdom
- Older people don't feel as cheated
- With age comes greater respect for health and life
- With age comes patience and contentment
- Older people are less psychologically threatened by disability and fatigue
- Older people can focus more on their own needs

Among perceived disadvantages:

- Older people's bodies are more worn down and less resilient
- Older people are more socially isolated
- Older people get less sympathy and are judged more harshly
- Older people are too compliant and patient[5]

Emotional Development

We like to believe that with age comes wisdom, and that we develop emotionally as we mature. You can see evidence of your emotional development in how you feel about yourself, care for yourself, and how you deal with others.

Mario sounds surprised that "at this point in my life, I'm actually very happy." He finds that he has become more self-assured and that he doesn't concern himself as much with the other people's opinions of him:

> Now I, pardon my Armenian, I don't give a flying fuck, you know? I just don't care. So I find that the older I've been getting and ... and my friends my own age say the same thing, most of us, you just get to a point where you realize life really just isn't about anything that anybody else thinks. It's about you. It's about what you think. You know, and who cares what anyone else thinks?

Mark feels as if he's "more comfortable with himself" and adds:

> Fifty-four meant, you know, never really having to, like, compare yourself to others that, you are who you are. And accepting who you are. You know? ... whether some people like that or not. And that's fine, you know. Some people might like me and some people may not like me and that's just me ... You almost don't care any more. This is who I am now.

Peter is finding that he loves himself now for the first time in his life:

> So I think it's ... it's almost like, you know, this is my journey. This is my way to accept myself, to love myself. Because probably I ... you know, and even with HIV [*laughs*] I don't think I would ... get to it.

Tim believes he takes much better care of himself:

> I think it's just experience. Living long enough that your experience teaches you things. Plus the HIV factor. And when you have, you know, it's ... it's common sense.

Anything that goes into your life is what's gonna determine how you look at life. It's all the pieces that create the puzzle.

George, too, finds that loving himself means making choices to do what he wants:

It's reassessment, it's not that people are doing less, people are doing more, but they're doing more of what they like to do instead of less of everything. Instead of doing everything, you know, I've got to be at the discos, I've got to be out, I've got to be here, I've got to be there. I've got to be at the leather clubs on Friday. I've got to do this, I've got to do that, I've got to do drugs. Now, I don't need to do all of that. Now I like to do this, I like to do that.

And Luis believes that since he cares more for himself he has more energy to show concern for others:

I think I'm doing more than I used to. Because what I'm doing now is more constructive. More valuable. What I was doing then, was partying, getting high. What I'm doing now, is volunteering, helping people. ... So, I'm doing more, or it's just the same, but in a different category.

As we age, opportunities for emotional and psychological growth abound. We can become more skilled at emotional regulation. We can learn to manage our emotions more effectively, allowing our feelings to pass rather than getting stuck in unpleasant emotions. Experience also helps us to manage conflict and to become more constructive in handling personal tensions. We can even develop richer and more complex emotional lives as we are able to experience feelings that are deeper and more nuanced than when we were younger. However, age alone does not produce personal growth. We must take an active role in our development in order for the opportunities for emotional and psychological growth to take hold.[6]

Emotional maturity at midlife involves developing a greater sense of self-esteem and an ability to care for yourself. When we love ourselves and treat ourselves right, we tend to take better care of others as well.

Evolving Spirituality

Another internal change that accompanies aging with HIV is an evolving sense of spirituality. You might find the subject of spirituality a difficult one. You are not alone. Histories of conflict with organized religions, many of which discriminate against gay people, leave gay men with ambivalent attitudes about religion. Tim was raised in a community of "bible thumpers" that condemned homosexuality. He rejected the religion of his family and moved to New York City to develop a positive self-image as a gay man. Today, he is not religious, but considers himself "spiritual."

George, too, doesn't practice Catholicism, but believes in a Higher Power.

Peter was not raised in a religious family. As an adult he studied Buddhism and meditates daily.

Joe's spirituality has grown over the years. He has educated himself across several traditions. His spiritual practices are a significant part of his daily self-care regimen. He explains:

> Usually I read a lot of things on … on spirituality and … there's nothing more profound for me than … spirituality, as a matter of fact.

Ronald faces many challenges. He is older, lives with HIV, is poor, is African American, and has been diagnosed with mental illness. He is not always comfortable reaching out to others for support. However, his faith is a significant source of strength for him:

> That's where my strength begins. I'm Baptist. Grew up in the Baptist church. Even though they still look down on people who are gay. And it seems they are afraid to mention the acronym AIDS in church. But there are good people there. And I need that kind of association to keep me balanced.

Although spirituality is not necessarily associated with healthy aging, a sense of faith can mitigate hardship, such as illness, lack of social support, and discrimination, as we get older.[7] Perhaps that is why spirituality is strongly associated with well-being among middle-aged and older people living with HIV[8] and why the men in this study most often defined themselves as not religious but spiritual.

I used to think that life was going to get easier as I grew older. I thought that with increased wisdom, personal growth, and professional development my relationships and work life would start to go smoothly and stress would be a thing of the past. Well, it hasn't worked out exactly the way I imagined. Yes, I have increased confidence and an ability to handle challenges, but life has not become the "smooth ride" that I imagined. New obstacles arise that I have never encountered, old problems keep coming up that I need to overcome, and, most surprisingly, my challenges have grown to meet my increased abilities. I am beginning to appreciate that my problems, still difficult at times, are opportunities for further development.

■ ASSIGNMENT ■

Evaluate your internal changes. Find photos of yourself at age 25, 35, and 45 (and every decade following until the present). If you cannot find a picture, create one in your mind's eye.

Place each photograph above a blank sheet of paper and answer the following questions on the corresponding page.

Self-knowledge: At age 25 (35, 45, etc.), how well do you know yourself? How often are you aware of what you are feeling (all of the time, sometimes, never?)? Do you know what you need and what is most important to you? Do you act on that knowledge effectively? Do you like yourself?

Self-care: Do you take good care of yourself? Manage your time well? Eat healthy foods? Sleep enough? Spend quality time with friends, relaxing, and having fun? Do you plan for your future? If you had one day to do anything you wanted at this age, how would you spend that day?

Relationships: Who are your best friends? How well do they know you? Do you share personal information with them? Rely on them? Let them rely on you? Are you satisfied with those relationships? What about your sex life and intimate relationships? If you could choose five people to spend the day with (from anywhere in the world, whom you know or don't know) who would you choose?

Spirituality: Do you have a spiritual practice, belief, or understanding? What gives your life meaning at this age? Are you compassionate toward others? How do you handle your own suffering? Do you connect with nature? Your breath? Music? Do you do service to others? Pray or meditate?

Compare the answers on each page: What do your responses tell you about your internal changes? Do you see a pattern? Do your circles get wider or smaller? Do you know and appreciate yourself more? What do your answers say about your priorities? Have you grown in ways that you like? What areas of your life could benefit from continued development?

Of course, change is not always for the better.

FAST FACT

In one study of middle-aged and older people living with HIV 29% of respondents demonstrated moderate or severe depression.[9]

Sometimes we regress or allow negative defenses (such as resentment, fear, pride, paranoia, and disdain) to fester and grow. Or we can become rigid, preventing ourselves from adapting internally to the changing environment—leading to increased isolation in old age. The next section will explore how the absence of adaptive internal change while aging with HIV can lead to getting stuck in midlife.

Summary

Congratulations!

You have successfully reviewed your life, acknowledged that aging means changing, considered the adaptations you have made, and evaluated your choices. It was quite an undertaking. Here's what Joe had to say about the work involved in adjusting to aging with HIV:

> So, the thing to do is pursue change and thrive with it and try to adjust with it. And that's a difficult thing to do for many people. Because once you sort of give up life and the thought of living and you prepare yourself to not being here anymore, to dying, and then suddenly you're told, "Don't think that way anymore. Scrap all that. And think this other way". It's not so easy. It's not so easy say for a man to be isolated on an island for sixty years and take him off the island and throw him into a future existence, where everything is different. Everything. Bar none.

Let's review. While you were caring for yourself and others, living through loss, and preparing for your mortality, aging approached without expectation. To cope with the challenges of aging with HIV, you first had to stop and acknowledge all the changes you have undergone. In the previous section you've identified nine areas in which aging has meant changing (the course of the AIDS epidemic, alterations in your body, changing friendship networks, developing a new place in the gay community,

95

developing a new attitude about sex, experiencing changing relationships, experiencing new roles in the family, developing a new approach to work, and internal changes). At this point, you should have a better understanding of how you've adapted to all these changes and assessed areas in which you need some help.

Remember, there is no one strategy of adaptation. This book is here to guide you through your *unique* path to optimal aging with HIV. Before we move on to the steps you can take to improve your life we need to identify areas in which you might have gotten stuck along the way.

SECTION II
ADAPTATION VERSUS STAGNATION

Introduction

In the previous section you have observed how aging means changing. You have identified nine areas of life in which aging with HIV requires you to adapt to change. And you've assessed your own adjustment, considering where you might have gotten stuck along the way.

The opposite of adaptation is stagnation: to stop developing and begin to decline. Health and mental health professionals consider the threat of stagnation to be the major challenge to adults at midlife. Gay men living with HIV may be at particular risk for stagnation in later life. Your diagnosis has already put much of your life on hold, and now that you're navigating middle age you have to catch up.[1]

RESEARCH REVIEW

The findings from my study of 15 gay men in middle age living with HIV helped me develop a theory of "adaptation versus stagnation." Adaptation vs. stagnation posits that gay men living with HIV have been knocked off course in their adaptation to aging, and that anticipated mortality, the magnitude of loss, and living with chronic illness have impeded their opportunities for gradual aging with a cohort of their peers. Adaptation vs. stagnation alludes to and expands on

---

Erikson's "generativity vs. stagnation." (See the Research Review box on page 77.) To experience continued growth in midlife and beyond we must use our knowledge and experience to aid in the development of future generations. "Adaptation vs. stagnation" helps us understand how gay men aging with HIV can meet the challenge of generativity: by regaining their position in the life course.

But these men can't just pick up where they left off and rejoin their life trajectory. While they've been aging with HIV/AIDS, life has gone on. HIV has evolved from a terminal illness to a chronic condition. The epidemic has devastated their social and personal lives. The gay community has changed. Their relationships to friends, family, and work have shifted. The importance of sex may have diminished for them and their expectation for intimate relationships has changed. And they have undergone dramatic alterations to their physical and emotional selves. Adapting to aging with HIV/AIDS involves adjusting to myriad changes on a new timeline.

The men I talked to proved that the threat of stagnation is real. In vivid, wistful detail—their words animate this entire book—they demonstrated an underlying urge to let life pass by, rather than define a new life course with the illness. They felt an overwhelming pull to live in past memories, to accept a shrinking kind of life, to deny the realities of aging, to lose interest in building friendship networks or intimate relationships, to shy away from paid and volunteer work, and to relinquish plans for the future.

Adaptation is an elusive concept. What is adaptive to one person in dealing with a problem at one point in time may be maladaptive to another, with a different issue, or at a different time. In fact, the men I interviewed did not display one single pattern of adaptation to aging with HIV. I cannot conclude from the interviews that this group is adjusting significantly well or poorly to the changes noted. Nor do I find that some individuals are coping significantly better than other respondents, or that, as a whole, individuals cope better with changes in one area over other areas.

What I did find was that adjustment to the changes associ-ated with aging with HIV is a multidimensional dynamic involving a spectrum of adaptation to each "field of change." "Adaptation versus stagnation," therefore, is a measure for evaluating how one is adjusting to aging with HIV on an indi-vidual level, and, more specifically, to each "field of change" involved. Meeting the challenge of adaptation versus stagna-tion means engaging in the ongoing process of adjusting to the changes associated with aging with HIV and redefining a new life course with the illness.[2]

Stagnation can be overwhelming, as it was for Joe when he thought about giving up entirely:

Then, the other question comes into point, what for? Why should I eat properly, exercise, stay active, not just lay back and wait to die, and go without medication and all these other things.

But stagnation can occur in subtle ways as well. Giving up on sex and dating, relinquishing career goals, not making new friends, avoiding social situations, getting stuck in old patterns with family, and relying on self-care strategies that are no longer successful can all be forms of stagnation. Even if you have been adapting well to many of the areas discussed in Section I, you may find that you are stuck in one or two others.

To help you evaluate your adaptation to aging with HIV, this section will pose four questions. Are you:

1. Learning from the past or living in the past?
2. Living within limitations or letting your world shrink?
3. Accepting yourself or getting stuck in your ways?
4. Living one day at a time or relinquishing a plan for the future?[3]

The following four chapters will help you answer these ques-tions and determine how well you are meeting the challenge of adaptation versus stagnation.

10

Learning from the Past or Living in the Past?

Entering Paul's apartment is like going through a time warp. The walls are filled with photos of Paul and his friends in their twenties and thirties. All of his artwork and decorations are from the 1970s and early 1980s. Even Paul's mustache, his clothes, and the way he styles his hair are reminiscent of the "clone" look of the 1970s. During an interview with Paul, I drew a line with one end in the past and one in the future (Fig. 10.1), and asked him to point to where he was. He said, "Right there. Oh, yeah, I'm in the past."

> **FAST FACT**
>
> Living in the past can be a challenge for gay men who wish to return to a pre-AIDS era and escape the omnipresent threat of living with HIV.[1] As the sociologist Kathy Charmaz explains, for people living with chronic illness, "when dull days replace vibrant years, the past can offer solace and refuge."[2]

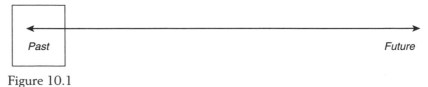

Figure 10.1

Living with HIV can reshape your sense of time. Life, as you knew it, may have stopped for you with your diagnosis, or the death of your closest friends. And memories of a fun-filled past can be comforting when illness and age make life seem dull. The need to learn from the past and reminisce can be challenged by the pull to live in the past and regret.

Living in the Past vs. Putting Things in the Past

Perhaps you have seen men like the ones Peter describes:

> **Sure I enjoyed going out and all that sort of thing, we all did. But I still ... I see people who are contemporaries and still think it's 1973. And I find it very sad.**

Or maybe you are one—a man whose friends think he's living in the past. But outward appearances can be deceiving. How do you know when you're stuck in the past?

The first question to ask yourself is whether you try to relive the past as a way to avoid stresses in the present. Tim finds that living in the past can be a way of actively avoiding the trauma of loss and the painful realities and stresses of life as a gay man living with HIV at midlife:

> **I think reverting back to barebacking was touching home base. Feeling the foundation. Visiting the past. Allowing myself to abandon everything.**

As Tim points out, his need to abandon everything gets in the way of accurately assessing and responding to his needs in the present. He puts himself and his partners at risk to have that moment of escape. When he comes back to the present, he feels regret and pain for what he has done.

A second question to ask yourself is whether overidentifying with a glorious past could impede your availability to opportunities that are being offered to you in the present. George dedicates a room in his two-room apartment to friends who died of AIDS. All four walls are covered with photos of friends who have died. George explains what makes the past so compelling for him:

> **Because the past was so brilliant, I mean the seventies were, I mean, you're too young to remember what they were like.**

> They were brilliant. I mean, no one set out to kill themselves.
> No one set out to catch a disease that was going to end their
> life. We were just having the time of our lives, and became
> very powerful politically. I mean, socially and politically, gay
> people were very powerful in the seventies. It was a very high,
> and I'm not talking about drugs, although drugs had a lot to
> do with it [*laughs*] but, I mean, without all that it was a very
> high time. It was very mind-expanding ... um ... broad expe-
> riences, happening with different people coming from all
> over. New York was a fascinating place to be because it all
> happened here.

Is George living in the past? George could potentially use that
room for storage, to develop a hobby, for guests, or for a new lover.
The psychic space George devotes to his past may be cluttering his
life and getting in the way of forming new relationships.

Yet the solution to living in the past is not putting things in the
past and shutting the door behind you. Jamie has a list of people,
places, and things that he has "put in the past." He no longer uses
drugs. He doesn't go to clubs. He doesn't date. He is not "in the
scene" anymore. He talks about no longer doing the things he used
to do:

> All that running around is no good for you. So most of the
> things that I used to do, all of that stuff is behind me now.

Jamie has put the past behind him, yet he has not found a way to
carry his needs, interests, and activities from the past into his life
today. He hasn't replaced what he has given up, and he is left with
a dull life. Rather than put your past interests behind you, you
must acknowledge what you gained from those experiences and
transform them into new tools that are usable and relevant to your
life today.

Reminiscing vs. Regret

The challenge is to learn from the past in order to live more fully
in the present and prepare for the future. This requires a flexible
ability to reflect on your past without getting mired in it.

RESEARCH REVIEW

Reminiscing is the process of thinking about your past experiences. Research in this area has demonstrated that reminiscing can have implications, both positive and negative, for healthy aging. Recalling memories of the past has three functions: life review, guidance, and emotional support. Life review allows us to synthesize positive and negative memories, assisting in our developing a continuous and evolving sense of self. We draw on past experiences for life lessons and guidance when coping with challenges in the present. And reminiscing can be a source of emotional regulation, affecting our social interactions. However, when the process of reminiscing is obsessive or escapist, it can have negative effects on our sense of self, emotional health, and the ability to interact effectively in the world.[3]

As Mark explains, reminiscing about the past is a normal part of growing older:

> I think you'd get that from anybody who is over fifty. You get to be a certain age and you reflect upon your life. We all do that.

Reminiscing serves an important role at midlife. We reflect on our past in order to gain perspective on our lives, as Hector does:

> Without the past it's not you. The past makes you who you are. It sort of molds me into who I am.

Arthur uses his memories to draw lessons from the past to apply to his present:

> I don't have any desire to reconstruct the past any more, but what I've been doing is trying to explain past events to show the bearing it may have on my present situation.

Finally, reminiscing can be a source of commonality with our peers. Joe bonds with members of his support group because they have shared memories:

> So I began to need people that were older to ... share with, because I no longer had that much in common with younger

people in that sense. And ... I lacked the perspective of an older person.

To have access to our memories, we cannot be overwhelmed with regret. We all have painful memories, experiences that we wish we could do over. We can learn from those experiences, too, as long as the pain of looking back is not so great as to prevent us from remembering. George speaks freely about his regrets, and how he must overcome them in order to grow:

> I made a lot of mistakes when I was young. They were foolish mistakes. I wish I had been smarter about money. I wish I was smarter about work, I wish I had been smarter about a lot of things, but what can I do now, you know, live and learn.

The first challenge of stagnation is becoming stuck in the past, either by trying to keep the past alive or by becoming overwhelmed with regrets. Optimal aging with HIV involves a flexible relationship to the past, having enough access to the past to reminisce and learn from the past, without becoming overwhelmed by it or unable to live in the moment and consider the future.

Can You Learn from the Past without Living in the Past?

How you answer this question can have implications across several areas of your life. You can deny the impact that developments in the treatment of HIV disease has had on your quality of life and life expectancy or accept them, disregard or adapt to physical changes, allow the memories of past friendships and loves to enrich your life or get stuck in them, remain committed to the sex life of your past or discover a fulfilling sex life today, get stuck in an old role in your family or develop new relationships with them, regret career decisions or increase your productivity, and relinquish an old view of yourself and allow for internal change and growth.

In my psychotherapy practice I work with people on the grieving process to help them learn from the past rather than live in the past. Mourning lost friends, family, and friends is only part of grief. Often people need assistance adapting to less tangible losses, including loss of community, physical limitations, youth, and missed opportunities. Sometimes we need help mourning the loss of what was never received, but longed for from parent, lovers, and friends. Moving out of the past often involves painful separation. In the long run grief benefits our emotional development and offers us the support and strength to deal with future challenges. Section III will offer you some guidance in your grieving process.

REFLECTION

Ask yourself the same question I asked Peter. Draw a line from the past, through the present, and into the future. Where would you place yourself?

Do you reminisce and remember old times by yourself or with friends?

When you think about the past, do you have regrets? If so, are they overwhelming?

Do you glamorize the past—was everything better then?

Are there people, places, and activities that you have put in the past? Have you ever reconsidered those things you have put behind you? Have you replaced them with new interests?

Now, reconsider the first nine chapters of this book. Reviewing the nine "fields of change" outlined individually (the AIDS epidemic, the gay community, your physical body, your role in the family, the world of work, your friendship networks, your sex life, intimate relationships, and internal changes), ask yourself whether you draw on your past experiences in each area to help you grow today, or whether you have gotten stuck in an old way of relating to one or more of these parts of your life.

In this chapter you have seen how past memories can be a source of support and guidance. You have also acknowledged that you can use the past as a refuge against the challenges of present life. At times the difference between learning from the past and living from the past can be difficult to distinguish. Only through rigorous honesty can you determine whether your perspective is aiding in your adaptation to aging with HIV or threatening stagnation. In the next chapter you will consider whether you are living within limitations or letting your world shrink.

11

Living within Limitations or Letting Your World Shrink?

Living with HIV involves coping with a number of limitations. The complications of living with illness over time can reduce your social involvement. Joe feels that the issues he faces, such as financial problems, physical challenges, not working with others, losses among friends and family, fewer recreational activities, and changing interests, have led to a "shrinking kind of life." But he also acknowledges how his tendency to isolate himself contributes to this dynamic:

> The less contact with people. The lower income. I mean by not working. The aging aspect as time goes on. The chronic illness and the things you've been through since it's been officially diagnosed. The hospitalization, operations, people around you passing away from illness. You can see the progression of illness in people that you spend time around. You kind of like reduce the people you're in contact with professionals, in terms of like clinicians, all kinds of medical people, and hospitals and therapies of all sorts. Other people involved in the same things that you are. Because of diminishing health in many cases your ability to do the things you used to do is no longer the same, so you have to cut back on all kinds of activities for a number of reasons. Age also makes a big difference. As you get older, as I mentioned, you require a different kind of attitude. You mature, or you gain a different kind of perspective on things, or I do, I can only speak

for myself. And a lot of this has led, with a lot of people, like myself, into a kind of isolation, because it's both imposed from the outside, as well as from your own personal kind of situation.

Living with illness, AIDS-related losses, and even aging can create real limitations. You may feel that you've learned to cope with these complications in your day-to-day life, but have you recognized the impact on your social involvement? It takes effort to counteract the shrinking kind of life that Joe describes. This chapter will help you evaluate whether you are living within limitations or letting your world shrink.

Fewer Options and Opportunities

Aging with HIV includes physical complications, financial limitations, and other challenges that reduce your options and opportunities. Mario knows the frustration that accompanies fewer choices:

> Well, I would say that honestly and realistically it has removed a lot of choices in life that would have been there had I not become positive. So I think that it has created a certain amount of frustration because there are things that you can't do that you may have been able to do had you not ever converted. And that's probably the only real big problem.

Patrick points out that the personal growth he has experienced as a result of living with HIV has come at a cost:

> Maybe I'm a better person because of AIDS. And I hate saying things like, in reality it was a blessing, you know? I just loathe and despise those kinds of comments. Cause … this is first and foremost a hideous experience and it should happen to nobody, you know?

In Section I we reviewed the physical changes to which you must adapt, including fatigue, diarrhea, pain, periodic illnesses, and lipodystrophy. Learning to live within these limitations is an integral part of managing chronic illness. You have made many changes to your life to adapt to physical limitations. George considers moving to an apartment on a lower floor; Patrick wears protective undergarments at times; Jamie occasionally uses a cane; Peter does temp work because it offers him flexibility when he is unwell.

Sometimes living within physical limitations is difficult to accept, as Mario explains:

> I have difficulty accepting that I have to slow down. I still try to multi-task but it doesn't work anymore. I have a much shorter fuse. I get spent quicker than I normally do. And taking that nap to me is accepting defeat.

But Luis knows that making those alterations is choosing to live:

> I mean, I could more or less, how do you put it, it could be any disease that you have in your body, you either live with the idea and put that in focus to yourself … or you choose to die. I don't choose to die. So I'm living comfortably with that disease.

You have also learned to live within financial limitations. Jamie has learned to stretch his disability check. Moving to the Bronx was difficult after a life in the "center of everything" in Manhattan, but now he appreciates the quiet. Ronald is glad to have an affordable apartment, but feels alienated in his building. Mario used to go to the theater, movies, and restaurants much more often, but now hunts for deals or free tickets through organizations he has joined. For George, the financial limitations that have accompanied his illness have been difficult to manage emotionally:

> Being HIV positive, having very limited resources, makes me feel very out of it.

FAST FACT

Middle-aged and older adults with HIV are almost eight times more likely to have negative or zero assets than their counterparts in the general population.[1] And financial limitations have been found to significantly and negatively affect social interaction among middle-aged and older people living with HIV/AIDS.[2]

Living within physical, financial, and other HIV and age-related limitations can gradually reduce your social involvement. You may find that you are spending less time out of the house or away from a bathroom, cutting back on paid or volunteer work, and engaging in fewer social and recreational activities. Ronald sees how living within limitations has affected the quality of his interactions:

> I see myself as being, at this point, isolated from the professional community, what as my friends were dedicated professionals.

George finds making new friends even more challenging because of his limitations:

> The idea of looking for new friends is difficult. Because I feel like, what does somebody that I find interesting, want to do with me who can't do anything? You know ... who can't ... spend money doing nice things. Or even not so great things but just regular things.

And Joe feels that the stigma of lipodystrophy has kept him from getting out more:

> I would probably be more out there if I didn't have physical detractions. And I'll cite particularly, facial atrophy ... It's an image problem also.

Some reduction in social interaction is expected with age. At midlife, age-related losses begin to occur among friends and family, retirement becomes an issue, and physical changes decrease our opportunities for social interaction. At the same time, our priorities shift and we tend to spend less time pursuing new social experiences, activities, and friends, and spend greater amounts of time with fewer people. For example, Jamie sees how aging has changed his interests and he doesn't want to go to the clubs, bars, and parties that were his main occupation in his youth. But, as Mario explains, the combination of changing interests and physical complications is manifest in much smaller circles of social involvement:

> But age is also a factor in terms of going out and leading a social life. Age factors in because, one, you're no longer interested in things you used to do. Your lifestyle has changed

with time. Your interests change. You pursue things other than what interested you, say, thirty years ago. So, the age factor, itself, is a factor in changing you and your attitude in general, but when that's coupled with a lot of chronic illness then you know, you have a problem.

Withdrawal

Whereas the limitations of aging with HIV can dramatically impact your social involvement, you can further constrict your world through withdrawal and isolation.

Joe knows that he plays a role in his shrinking kind of life, because he has always had a tendency to isolate. But now he sees that it has gotten to an extreme:

> **The reason I need therapy is that I am a loner and I've become even more of a loner. And I need someone to talk to. My muscles turn to stone from the tension.**

Ronald has always considered himself an outgoing person. Although he would prefer to "be of service" to others, he has become withdrawn in response to the stigma of living with HIV:

> **I would rather do a service for someone, rather than shun someone in order to keep my confidentiality. But I find myself having to shun people and in those cases those people don't understand why I do so and I cannot tell.**

Jamie used to be very socially active, but now he feels little interest in going out of the house:

> **Yeah, if I wasn't going out to do something, no, I wouldn't go out. That's why a lot of people that used to invite me to parties don't invite me no more 'cause I don't never show up ... When I was younger, all I wanted to do is party, party, party, now that I'm older, things change. I don't feel the same. I prefer to stay home.**

And George believes that he is *mostly* content on his own:

> **Well that's why I'm pretty happy ... I'm pretty happy by myself ... I'm not always happy by myself.**

Living within physical, financial, and other limitations may have reduced the number and frequency of your social interactions. Additionally, changing interests and priorities can further impact your friendships and activities. As Joe, Jamie, and George point out, you can participate in a shrinking kind of life by withdrawing from the world.

Locus of Control

One way to figure out whether you are living within limitations or letting your world shrink is to ask yourself: "Who is in control?" Are you adapting to physical, financial, and other limitations that are unchangeable or does the power to expand your social involvement lie within you? When asked whether the constrictions Ronald refers to are imposed from within or without, he explains:

> I would say 80 percent is imposed from without, because the virus has taken 99 percent of my friends away. They have passed on. I see myself as being, at this point, isolated from the professional community, what as my friends were dedicated professionals.

RESEARCH REVIEW

The research on HIV over 50 demonstrates the ambiguity between living within limits and letting your world shrink. There is evidence that middle-aged and older people living with HIV experience a dramatic decline in social involvement, which results in "fragile networks of social support."[3] In contrast, gay men and other groups of people living with HIV over age 50 report flexibility and resilience in response to the impact age, loss, and stigma have had on their social networks, and that they seek out and rely on HIV-positive people who offer empowerment, commonality, and inspiration.[4] One possible explanation for this apparent contradiction lies in the concept of a locus of control. People with a greater sense of internal locus of control, who feel that they have greater influence over their life, have better health and well-being at midlife[5] and a better adjustment to illness in general.[6] People with a greater internal sense of self-efficacy may be more able to live within the limits of HIV- and age-related losses while counteracting a shrinking kind of life by rebuilding satisfying social networks.

In my psychotherapy practice I work with people to help them determine whether they have control over a given situation, and, if so, how they can effect change in their lives. You cannot stop by just acknowledging the real limitations of aging with HIV. Once you accept what you are powerless over, you can determine what is within your control. The serenity prayer offers clarity to many who seek guidance in distinguishing between powerlessness and control:

God, grant me the serenity to accept the things I cannot change, courage to change the things I can, and wisdom to know the difference.[7]

In Section III we will discuss more tools you can use to work within your limitations to determine where your agency lies.

Confronting a Shrinking Kind of Life

Once you see where you have the opportunity to effect change, you must be willing to take the action, and the risk, to expand your limitations and confront a shrinking kind of life. You may feel more content on your own, like George. However, this does not absolve your responsibility to remain active and involved. Perhaps, like Jamie, age and illness make you feel more vulnerable outside your home. Or, like Ronald, the stigma of aging with HIV has heightened an old tendency to isolate. A shrinking kind of life can sneak up on you, and if you are not vigilant, you may find it too easy to withdraw. But if you give up on the world, the world will give up on you.

Joe talks about the work he must put into maintaining his quality of life:

> Because I know to maintain any quality of life you have to do some input. You have to eat, you have to exercise, you have to keep your mind active, you have to partake in activities, you know, functions, you have to care about other people, and try to integrate your life with other people.

Luis recognizes that physical changes and changing priorities have created losses in his life, but he also sees the need to replace old interests with new ones:

> I think I'm doing more than I used to. Because what I'm doing now is more constructive. More valuable. What I was doing then was partying, getting high. What I'm doing now is volunteering, helping people. So, I'm doing more, or it's just the same, but in a different category.

Can You Live with Limitations without Letting Your World Shrink?

This question can be answered by examining the nine changes identified in Section I, including your adaptation to the losses associated with HIV, changes in your body, your relationship to the gay community, your sex life and intimate relationships, your family involvement, your work life, and even how you respond to the internal changes that have accompanied aging with HIV.

REFLECTION

Do you relate to Joe's comment about his shrinking kind of life?

What are the limitations that you face?

Has your social involvement gotten smaller over the years?

How much control do you have over your shrinking life?

Have you attempted to add new friends and activities into your life? If not, what gets in the way?

> What do you think your life will be like in 10 years if you make no changes to your social interaction today?
>
> Now, review the first nine chapters of the book again and ask yourself whether you have been living within limitations in each "field of change," or whether you have been letting your world shrink in one or more of these areas of your life.

In this chapter you have observed how losses of friends, physical challenges, retirement, financial limitations, and changing interests can lead to a smaller scope of activities and social interaction. But you have also seen that you can make matters worse by withdrawing from the world. You should have a better sense of where you have control to create change and how you can balance contentment with being on your own with the benefits of having an active life. In the next chapter you will further explore the challenge of adaptation versus stagnation by asking yourself whether you are accepting yourself or getting stuck in your ways.

12

Accepting Yourself or Stuck in Your Ways?

One of the advantages of aging with HIV is that you become more comfortable with yourself. Hopefully, as you have gotten older you have developed greater self-awareness and self-acceptance. Although these are the positive developments of aging, sometimes it is difficult to acknowledge when "knowing yourself" is really just an excuse for being set in your ways. Continued growth throughout midlife and beyond is central to optimal aging with HIV.[1] This chapter will help you examine whether you are accepting yourself or getting stuck in your ways.

Accepting Yourself

At midlife we have a much better sense of ourselves. We know who we are, what we like, and how we are going to react in situations. This developed self-awareness can result in a greater appreciation of ourselves, reduced insecurity with others, and greater confidence.

Mark was an insecure kid. He was uncomfortable about his appearance and shy. Today, he is a handsome, outgoing, middle-aged man who doesn't care as much about what others think about him. As Peter has gotten older he, too, has grown to accept a great deal about himself. He accepts his sexual orientation more than he ever has. He accepts his HIV status and is no longer as traumatized as he was by it. He accepts his anxiety and has learned to cope with it better. And he accepts aging, which, he feels, allows him to take better care of himself:

> Ever since I turned 50 ... it's sort of a ... not a ... resignation in a bad way but sort of an acceptance of being 50 and now it's about maintaining stuff. Strength and stamina and flexibility and stuff like that.

George has grown to accept and like himself more. He has lost a great deal of weight recently and is beginning to consider dating for the first time in over a decade:

> But I keep saying to myself even if I stay without a relationship, I'm very happy for what I did because I feel wonderful about myself.

But George recognizes that although he thinks about dating, he makes no effort to meet someone new. He has a set routine and his schedule tells him when to eat, walk the dog, and call his friends. George knows himself well, does what he likes, and is content on his own, but he leaves little room for romance.

Getting Stuck in Your Ways

It can be easy to slip into a comfortable routine when you accept yourself. You develop certain patterns and daily rituals. You see the same people, participate in the same activities, and go to the same places on a regular basis, because you know who you like and what you enjoy doing. But getting stuck in your ways can leave little room for growth in midlife. Mark describes how he can get set in his ways:

> You know, you get to a certain cycle and habits and behaviors. I mean I certainly am aware of how I've gotten older in my likes, dislikes ... things that I have no patience for that I used to have patience for.

And Mario recognizes how his habits have gotten rigid with age:

> You're not so quick to just leave everything behind and start over in your middle age as, you know, when you're younger you go, oh I'll get new friends. You know, so I'm sort of locked in.

During our entire two-hour interview, Hector did not turn off the television, he just turned down the volume. He told me the series of shows he watches every day. He has a few activities that he enjoys, an HIV support group that he attends, and friends he speaks to on the phone, but he admits that he spends most of his time in front of the television.

Are these men just doing what they want to do or getting stuck in their ways?

Living with illness can make this question a complicated one. Sometimes your physical health makes life change impossible. You just don't have the energy or ability to do anything more. At others times you may feel better, but wonder how long it will last. HIV-related illnesses can seem to emerge suddenly with no explanation. You may be concerned that changing your routine, trying something new, or challenging yourself may cause stress or have an impact on your health. The only way to know whether you are accepting the status quo and stagnating or just taking good care of yourself is to test your fear, to gradually and safely try a small change, and to evaluate the outcome.

For Patrick the question of whether to accept the status quo or strive for more at this stage of his life is existential. He wonders if he should try to make up for time lost to HIV or just take it easy:

> A crucial piece of this is that I am 55 and there are those things about 55 that make you want to say, oh just relax, you know? Just, I mean, life, what is it? If you live to be a hundred you got 45 more years, maybe you should just really enjoy yourself, you know? But on the other hand because that was snatched out of my life in my late 30s and throughout my 40s, I'm scrambling to have those experiences that I should have had when I was younger. You know, but since I didn't have them, so I'm conflicted between being 55 and going, well gee you're 55, you know, it's hard to get out of bed, just relax! Enjoy your life, you know? Don't work so hard. And then this other part that's still hungry.

Patrick's concern is common for gay men who find that they have lived longer than they ever expected. How *can* you live with HIV has evolved into how do you *want* to tackle midlife and beyond?

Continued Growth in Midlife and Beyond

Not only is continued growth in middle age an integral part of healthy aging, but challenging yourself is also a way to survive and thrive with HIV. For Patrick the threat of stagnation was a life-threatening challenge that had to be confronted in order to live:

> I need to challenge myself. The reason I feel that I may be being challenged, is that I could not let that dominate my life. I had to seek other avenues. Because that is essential for one's survival. I'm not sure how successful I have been. I've been successful in recognizing that. I think that I am working very diligently in creating new avenues.

For Arthur, there is no conflict between accepting himself and continuing to grow. After living with HIV for many years his viral load suddenly increased and his doctor recommended beginning antiviral therapy. Arthur believes that accepting this new reality and challenging himself to evolve go hand-in-hand:

> I have to also learn to accept a lot of things. And I cannot. I have to evolve. Well, you know, I am no longer … Well, things have changed that I now have to take a cocktail, and I just accept it and it's another form of evolution. And that evolution is, because of accepting that and realizing that it is, that there's no such thing as immortality. I'm embracing life as it is and challenging myself.

Peter doesn't believe he is restarting where he left off, but rather believes that he is creating a new path for himself with the virus:

> I'm a survivor and I'm gonna flourish too…. it's interesting, I think that it's not a matter of reclaiming or restarting where I left off, but fulfilling more of my life. My potential.

For these men living with HIV, continuing to grow at midlife is not an option, but an imperative. To challenge themselves, to evolve, and to flourish are integral to their survival, and stagnation must be avoided at all costs.

FAST FACT

Stagnation at midlife can lead to self-absorption, feeling little connection to others, isolation, and a lack of any sense of meaning in life.[2] Generativity counteracts stagnation through the act of giving of oneself to the next generation. For participants in one study of adult development, being involved in generative activities, such as acting as a consultant, guide, mentor, or coach, tripled the chances that their 70s would be a time of joy and not of despair.[3]

Research on aging tells us that generativity is the primary strategy to confront stagnation at midlife. Generativity means thinking beyond yourself and considering what you have to offer to others. Generativity is evident in Ronald's desire to be part of a process of bettering the world, a challenge that he knows will outlive him:

I was saying that being gay presents a challenge of its own and I'm not sure that a gay man or woman can truly overcome those challenges in one lifetime. I think it may be necessary to work on a problem to begin to see a possible solution. Do what you can working toward that solution. And then leave it to someone ... the next younger generation coming.

Luis demonstrates generativity in his attempt to give of himself and help his family member to resolve their conflicts with one another:

I just want to at least give 'em something so they could remember me, you know?' Cause if I go away, at least that'll bring 'em together. If it's for criticism or laughter or whatever ... But I would like to also give of myself and not just freeze.

And Tim shows that he wants to be generative by passing things on to the next generation:

Again, for my friends that are dead ... but it's not for me, it's for the future as my friends did it for me, I want to do it for them. I want to make the future better for ... the people, whether they're related to me or not that follow me.

You can be generative through involvement with children, mentoring young adults, volunteering to assist and educate others, or any activity that keeps you participating in the larger society, caring for others, and passing on your wisdom. Section III will discuss in greater depth strategies to remain generative in midlife and beyond.

Can You Accept Yourself without Getting Stuck in Your Ways?

You have had to accept a great deal while aging with HIV, including changes in your body, loss, retirement, your role in the family, your relationship, and even your priorities and interests. But accepting yourself does not mean accepting the status quo, but rather using your self-awareness to help you identify your strengths and weaknesses and determine where you need to challenge yourself for further growth.

REFLECTION

Do you have a set routine of activities, interactions, and places you go?

How much opportunity do you give yourself for new experiences and growth? Why?

In what ways are you generative?

Once again, review the first nine chapters and consider your patterns in each area of life: Are you accepting of yourself or getting stuck in your ways?

You have seen the subtle ways in which being comfortable with yourself can slip into getting stuck in your ways, that accepting yourself at midlife does not mean avoiding opportunities for growth, and how remaining involved in generative activities can help you avoid the threat of stagnation. In the next chapter you will consider the following question: Are you living one day at a time or avoiding plans for the future?

13

One Day at a Time or Avoiding the Future?

The final question in the challenge of adaptation versus stagnation is whether you are living one day at a time or avoiding the future. We know that living one day at a time is a healthy and adaptive strategy. This life approach is recommended for people recovering from addictions and compulsions, anxiety disorders, people with physical challenges, in healthy aging, and for anyone who wants to live more fully in the present. However, even good medicine can be overused and abused, and we can use this healthy approach as an excuse to avoid planning. This chapter will help you find your optimal path toward aging with HIV by considering the following question: Are you living one day at a time or are you avoiding the future?

One Day at a Time

People in recovery from alcoholism, substance abuse, or other addictions know the value of living one day at a time. Expectations about the future can quickly lead to overwhelming anxieties and resentments, triggers for compulsive behaviors. Living one day at a time means focusing on the present, staying sober for today, and not getting caught up in what the future might bring. As people recovering from alcoholism have learned, "First, we try living in the now just in order to stay sober—and it works. Once the idea has become a part of our thinking, we find that living life in 24-hour segments is an effective and satisfying way to handle many other matters as well."[1]

You can see the effects of living one day at a time in your approach to HIV. When you first learned your HIV status you may have become overwhelmed with worries about the future: How will you cope with the news? How will you tell your partners, friends, and family? What if you become ill? Will you die from HIV disease? When you adapted to your status you became less overwhelmed about what could happen and learned that these concerns could be dealt with on a daily basis.

Mario used to worry about his health and financial security. Today, he sees how living one day at a time has improved his emotional well-being:

> **I take every day as it comes. I try to live in the moment. I have my moments when I worry about this. I worry about financial security. Yadayadayada. But I also know that worrying doesn't solve anything, it just makes you worry.**

As we age we learn that living one day at a time enriches our lives. Sure, there are things to be concerned about—illness, physical limitations, financial challenges, and mortality. But if we project ourselves into the future we can spoil the precious time we have left. "Carpe diem: Seize the day, but only one day at a time," writes Dr. George E. Vaillant in *Aging Well*. "The past and the future can be for the moment ignored."[2] Living one day at a time allows us to make the most of the time we are given.

Mark believes that living one day at a time is part of the wisdom of age:

> **The wisdom of age, if I can say I have any wisdom, is you realize the future is now. You get up in the morning, god forbid you could get hit by a bus tomorrow. You have to take each day as it comes because the best laid plans, you know it's cliché, cliché, cliché, you know you can plan all you want, but it's not going to work out that way. I think that for most people life is not what you plan. You can't plan.**

Living one day at a time involves accepting where you are today without beating yourself up for past mistakes or agonizing about the future. No matter what your age, health status, recovery status, or spiritual orientation, you can benefit from working on what immediately faces you, taking small steps, and making the most of the day—so, then, why do I include "living one day at a time" in the challenges of adaptation versus stagnation? Because even though this slogan is an adaptive tool to deal with HIV, aging, and life in general, it can be used to avoid necessary planning for the future.

Planning for the Future

Living longer with HIV means having to reintegrate the possibilities of aging into middle and older age and planning a future given up to the virus. As Tim explains:

> Yeah, well, before, I didn't think about the future, but I think about it now, you know? Not that it loses my sleep or lowers my T cells, you know what I'm trying to say? But I do think of it, you know, where am I gonna be 10 years from now.

Perhaps, like Tim, you gave up planning for the future when you learned that you had HIV. Now that you have realized that you are living longer than you ever expected, you have to think about the future. Since you are reading this book, I know that you are concerned about aging. Planning for life into old age involves thinking ahead to the future and anticipating your financial, social, and physical needs. But planning for the future also involves having a vision of yourself and what you want out of your life.

For George, planning for the future includes thoughts of entering another relationship:

> I mean at 58 or 59, whatever it will be, I will put myself back on the market again as someone who's ready to hang out and maybe find some kind of sexual ... relationship where I feel confident in myself and my own body is not an embarrassment for me.

Planning for the future for the first time since his diagnosis, Mark is rethinking his choices in several areas in his life, including his career and where he wants to live:

> I'd say, in the past year, two years that I've been thinking about it. And I ... actually, James, I have no idea. I don't

know if I want to write a book. I wouldn't know the first thing about it. I don't know if I want my real estate license. I don't know if I want to buy a house ... and fix it up and flip it. I don't know if I want to go work in a bookstore somewhere. Be on Cape Cod or go down to Florida for the winter and work in something or ... I have no idea of where I'm going.

If you don't have a plan for the future you could find yourself directionless in middle age and ill-prepared for the challenges of later life. In Section III we dedicate a step to help you plan for your newfound future.

Can You Live One Day at a Time and Still Plan for the Future?

Both planning for the future and living one day at a time are integral to healthy aging with HIV. It can be difficult to distinguish which approach is most adaptive. And sometimes there is only a subtle difference between the two, as Peter demonstrates:

Planning for the future means showing up today. I don't know what the future holds, but there will be a future. And that's good, but it doesn't interest me as much as being in the present.

So, how do you know whether you are living one day at a time or avoiding the future? The answer to this difficult question lies in acknowledging whether fear of aging, illness, and mortality impedes your ability to envision a future.

How you feel about aging can have an effect on your plan for the future. Internalized stigma, ageist attitudes, and negative preconceptions about aging can make us deny the reality that we are growing older. Jamie, for example, doesn't want to think about getting older. He doesn't like the way he looks now, and anticipates that as he gets older he will become more isolated from his social life. He cannot see himself aging into a respected elder or a "grand dame" but is limited by his distaste for "bitter, old queens."

Patrick, on the other hand, is proud of getting older:

I kind of feel like, you know, you're lucky you get to be old.

His attitude about aging helps him to think about growing older without fear. He is able to think in the long-term because he is not put off by the thought of aging. In Section III we will discuss strategies for confronting ageist attitudes in yourself and others.

Another obstacle to planning for people living with HIV is anticipated illness, as Joe explains:

> Everyone likes to have a goal, but it becomes difficult for people with chronic illness to be goal oriented in that sense. Necessarily, some people it wouldn't let it faze them, they would pursue their objectives anyway. And others, I mean, I have a problem with that also. I wonder why sometimes. Why am I putting all this effort into all of this?

Uncertainty about your health can make you question whether you can achieve your goals, or whether it is better to just put them aside for today. But just as the enjoyment of sex includes not only the orgasm, but everything leading up to it, so, too, can the path toward accomplishing a goal be as satisfying as the outcome. When you let fear of anticipated illness unnecessarily restrict your vision for the future you deny yourself the opportunity to engage in that journey.

Finally, your sense of mortality directly impacts your ability to imagine and plan for a future. As Patrick explains, if you don't believe that you are going to live to old age, there's no reason to plan for the future:

> Healthy denial. I'm not denying that I'm not taking my Coletra every day. Or denying to the extent that I don't know what my blood sugar is. But, you know, when two people die from HIV and they are, one was 49 or 50 and the other was my age, he was probably 55, it just sort of startles me, jolts me back to the reality that this is not an impossibility, and it makes me question all of my career trajectories. Oh, I'm working to become a therapist and working to do this and that, and I'm not collecting social security disability and I'm thinking that I'll be getting my social security when I'm 67 like everybody else, and these things come along and I think, you're not, you're not, Patrick. You might get sick and something is going to happen in the next few years. And you should be going to Spain and eating at a café in Barcelona or you should be renting a convertible in Arizona.

Planning for the future means integrating hope with the realities of mortality. People are still dying of AIDS-related illnesses and no one is guaranteed a long life. However, advances in the treatment of HIV disease have made it possible to live with HIV into middle and older age. You must rethink your longevity and relinquish old expectations of mortality to create a future with HIV. Perhaps Luis is acknowledging the tenuous balance between accepting mortality and planning for the future when he talks about "applying to get into eighty":

> **The idea is to not to lose focus. To get every knowledge that I could possibly get. I mean, it's never too late. It could be 60, it could be 70, it could be 80. If others could … have done it, I could do it too, you know? I'm applying to get into 80. You know, with HIV. My dear friend next to me. And hopefully they'll find a cure.**

There is only a subtle difference between living one day at a time and avoiding the future. But given the importance of planning for middle and older age, you must reevaluate your fears of aging and previously held conceptions of your mortality to create a healthy balance between these two approaches. As you consider the following questions you can see how your choice to live one day at a time or plan for the future has been expressed in your attitude toward your physical changes, work, and relationships.

REFLECTION

How much do you rely on the slogan, "one day at a time?"
Does this preclude your plans for the future?
Are you afraid of growing older? Why or why not?
Do concerns about illness get in the way of your vision for the future?
Have you let yourself consider the possibility of living with HIV into old age?
Once again, review the first nine chapters and consider your patterns in each area of life: Are you living one day at a time or avoiding the future?

Now that you have answered the four questions of adaptation versus stagnation you are ready to move on to the steps toward optimal aging with HIV. But first, let's review what you have accomplished so far.

Summary

You now understand the theory of adaptation versus stagnation and are able to apply it to your life. You see how the threat of mortality, living with illness, and the loss of your friends and community to AIDS have knocked you off your life course. To get back on track you must adapt to changes in the nine areas discussed in Section 1. But rejoining life is not easy, and the threat of stagnation is real. You can get caught up in living in the past, let your world shrink, become stuck in your ways, and avoid plans for the future.

The difference between adapting and stagnating is often difficult to distinguish, and sometimes healthy strategies, including learning from the past, living within limitations, accepting yourself, and living one day at a time, can be misused to avoid the challenges of aging with HIV. To see where you could have gotten stuck along the way, you have had to complete a rigorous self-examination, considering your approach to life across all nine areas of change.

The challenge of adaptation versus stagnation is universal, but your approach is unique to you. And you may be adapting to changes in one area of life while stagnating in others. You have also become aware of the subtle differences between adaptation and stagnation, and that what was once an adaptive approach for you can become maladaptive at a different time. The four questions posed to you in this section have been your guide in this exploration. You may want to review these questions periodically to ensure that you are remaining flexible and adaptive in your approach to aging with HIV.

With this knowledge, acquired from a deep and thoughtful review of your life, you are ready to take the 10 steps toward optimal aging with HIV.

SECTION III

TEN STEPS TO OPTIMAL AGING WITH HIV

Introduction

In the first two sections of this book you looked back—reviewing and evaluating your adaptation to aging with HIV. This third section will offer you guidance on how to move forward, with flexibility and strength, to make the most of your current life and meet the challenges ahead.

Before you begin your journey, I have two pieces of advice:

First: **Embrace life**. Some gay men have become overwhelmed by the losses that have accompanied aging with HIV. They have withdrawn from the world and have no plans for the future. They live life as if they are waiting for something to happen. Others, though, recognize that life is for the living.

You are the only person who can make things happen in your life, one day at a time. Start today. Let yourself fantasize. Listen to your dreams. Talk with other people about goals. Make a list of things you want to do with your life. What steps do you need to take to achieve those goals? Identify one task on which you can begin working right now. Give yourself permission to live.

Second: **Keep it simple**. Don't make your life more complicated than it needs to be. As you take the 10 steps toward optimal aging consider the most obvious obstacles that are getting in your way, and find the simplest solutions to removing them. In this section there will be very few assignments, questions to answer, and references to the literature. You've already done all that. This section will present some basic steps you can take to improve your life. Try not to get overwhelmed by any of the suggestions presented.

Take them one at a time. Make small changes and observe the result before you move on to the next step. Remember, you can always revisit an issue when you're ready to do more.

The advice given here may seem simplistic. These are written as "first steps" in your unique path. The resources listed at the end of each step will offer guidance and in-depth exploration of each theme.

RESEARCH REVIEW

My in-depth study of gay men living with HIV in late middle age identified the unique constellation of changes that we explored in Section I. In Section II, we examined the theoretical and practical challenge of adapting versus stagnating in the face of these changes. This section will now focus on the nine "contributing factors" that can enhance or impede optimal aging. These contributing factors emerged from the hours of interviews with the men in my study as they talked about historical factors, internal resources, resilience, external resources, physical health, AIDS stigma, feelings about aging, mortality, and sense of agency.[1]

Using these factors as a foundation, I have incorporated research on HIV and aging as well as my clinical training and experience as a psychotherapist to develop the strategy for optimal aging with HIV that forms the core of this book. This 10-step model will help you map your unique path to health and well-being at midlife and beyond.

Your goal now is to reassess, reengage, and rebuild. This section will present a 10-step strategy to help you in that process. These tools should help you begin your journey to optimal aging with HIV right now.

Step 1

Care for Your Physical Health

Why Is It Integral That You Care for Your Physical Health?

Joe does not need to conduct a major research study to know that illness can make you isolated and depressed, and that isolation and depression can make you physically ill. He knows from experience that it is essential to do the most you can to maintain your health:

Because of diminishing health in many cases your ability to do the things you used to do is no longer the same, so you have to cut back on all kinds of activities for a number of reasons.

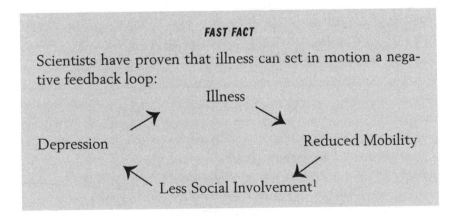

FAST FACT

Scientists have proven that illness can set in motion a negative feedback loop:

Illness

Depression

Reduced Mobility

Less Social Involvement[1]

But aging with HIV is new territory and little is known about how HIV interacts in an aging body.

As we identified in Chapter 2, as you age with HIV, your health care can become more complicated. First you had to adapt to living with HIV and now you must adjust to the slow progression of aging. Sometimes it is difficult to distinguish between the symptoms of age and HIV. And years of taking HIV medications can cause various changes in your body. Older bodies can react to medications differently than younger ones. And treatments for age-related complications, such as heartburn or cardiovascular health, can interact with HIV medications. Adapting to the physical changes of aging with HIV means reinvesting in your physical care, similar to how you adapted to caring for your body when you learned your HIV status.

How Do You Care for Your Physical Health Now?

Much like in the early days of the epidemic, midlife and older people living with the virus have to draw from what is known from many sources as well as from their own experience to determine what is best for their physical health.

Here are our recommendations for caring for your physical health.

Partner with Your Doctor

Your doctor's job is to listen to you and then, using his or her medical knowledge, offer you advice and help you take care of yourself. To do this, the two of you must communicate effectively.

TIPS TO GET THE MOST OUT OF YOUR VISIT WITH YOUR DOCTOR

- Arrive at appointments with a list of the concerns that you want to discuss.
- Tell your doctors everything, even if you think they will disagree. The more your doctor knows you, the more effectively he or she can help.
- If you don't understand something your doctor is telling you (or if you disagree with something he or

---

she says), say so. This is an opportunity to enhance your understanding of your own body and for your doctor to understand you.

- Bring a list of your medications, including over-the-counter medications, herbal medications and vitamins; meds you've stopped taking on your own; and medications you've been prescribed by other physicians. There may be drug interactions. For example, many over-the-counter and prescription antacids (Prilosec®, Prevacid®, Pepcid®, Zantac®, Tums®) can interfere with atazanavir (Reyataz®). Blood pressure medication (amlodipine) can interact with HIV medications. Be sure to talk to your HIV doctor before using these medications.
- Make a note of any refills needed.
- Ask for copies of your test results.
- Coordinate your care. Let your HIV doctor know which doctors you're seeing and bring copies of your reports and results.
- Write down (or have your doctor write down) any recommendations.

If you find that you cannot work effectively with your doctor and that it hinders your trust, it may be time to find a new physician.

Stay Informed

There may have been a time when you knew all there was to know about HIV, but now there is so much more information. Knowledge about HIV is expanding at a rapid pace and new research is constantly emerging that forces us to reconsider previous ideas and assumptions. Although you may not be able to know everything out there, you can still stay informed. The resources at the end of this section will point you to some excellent sources of current research, recommendations, and advances.

See Your Doctor Regularly

How often you see your HIV doctor needs to be customized by you and your doctor. A good rule of thumb is, if you are stable and without complications on antiviral medications, you should see your doctor and have blood tests approximately every 3–4 months.[2] People whose virus is not well controlled or who have multiple medical problems may need to see their doctor more frequently. Talk to your doctor about what schedule is most appropriate for you.

Get Screened

As we age, the chances of developing other HIV- and non-HIV-related illnesses increase. You and your doctor should routinely discuss general preventive health measures. The following is a general recommended schedule of exams and preventive measures:

- Annual sexual health assessment and counseling, including STD screening, syphilis screening, and HIV prevention
- Assessment and counseling for tobacco and substance use including alcohol
- Annual mental health screening, including depression and cognition
- Eye exam, including glaucoma screening, every 2 years beginning at age 40 and annually after age 60, but more frequently depending on the findings, other underlying problems (such as diabetes), or if your T cell count is <50
- Yearly body mass index (BMI), a measure of your height and weight
- Annual blood pressure check after age 40, more frequently if you have high blood pressure
- Cholesterol and blood sugar testing (see comorbid conditions below)
- Colon cancer screening starting at age 50, earlier if there is a family history
- Counseling about prostate cancer starting at age 50, sooner if you are African-American or have a family member with early prostate cancer
- Annual anal cancer screening (talk to your doctor about what kind of screening is appropriate for you)

- Annual digital rectal exam beginning at age 50
- Annual skin cancer exam
- Annual tuberculosis screening
- Immunizations: influenza annually, hepatitis A and B series, pneumococcal polysaccharide (as indicated based on your circumstances), and tetanus booster every 10 years

The timing of testing and follow-up are determined by your doctor depending on the findings, your medical history, family history, and other risk factors.

Take Your Medications Exactly as Prescribed

HIV medications can quickly stop working (i.e., "develop resistance") if they are not taken properly. That is, if you miss or skip doses or take only some of your pills, if you are taking other medications that reduce their absorption, or if you do not follow the food requirements, you may not have enough medication in your system to suppress HIV. Sometimes taking medications can be emotionally stressful, a daily reminder of HIV. If you believe your feelings are interfering with following a medication regimen talk to your doctor or counselor.

Monitor Comorbid Conditions

There are several conditions (outlined in Section I) that affect middle-aged and older people living with HIV at greater rates. For example, if you have diabetes or heart disease, your target levels of cholesterol and blood pressure should be lower than that of the general population. The treatment guidelines for these problems are the same as for the non-HIV-infected population. Therefore, your doctor will recommend lifestyle changes, such as quitting smoking, exercising, weight management, and changing your diet, and he or she will monitor blood tests more frequently. Because of HIV, your doctor may discuss switching away from antiviral medications that are associated more closely with cholesterol and high sugar levels and starting other medications to treat these conditions.[3] For example, switching from a protease inhibitor-based regimen to a nevirapine-based regimen may improve your cholesterol levels.

Or switching protease inhibitors, such as from lopinavir/ritonavir (Kaletra®) to atazanavir (Reyataz®), may also improve your cholesterol or blood sugar levels. You should have a frank conversation with your doctor about adding medications to lower cholesterol versus making changes to your HIV regimen, paying close attention to your cardiovascular risks and previous HIV regimens. For example, if you have previously taken nevirapine (and if your HIV was not completely suppressed), if you restart it, you may risk your viral load becoming detectable and developing resistance.

Bone loss (osteoporosis and osteopenia) appears to be more prevalent among HIV-infected people. Several factors can contribute to bone loss, including duration of HIV infection, use of corticosteroids, low testosterone, sedentary lifestyle, smoking, and some HIV medications.[4] However, at this time the routine measuring of bone density ("DEXA scan") is not recommended.[5] Those at risk or who have bone loss should minimize modifiable risk factors (stop smoking, minimize alcohol consumption, and increase exercise) and discuss calcium and vitamin D supplementation, testing, and other interventions with their doctor.[6]

Consider the Impact of Lipodystrophy

Lipodystrophy can cause emotional strain. If you are distressed by the appearance of facial wasting, a buffalo hump, or a protuberant belly ("protease paunch" or "crix belly") you may want to consider treatment options. Counseling may help you develop the emotional coping skills and face the restigmatizing impact of lipodystrophy. There are also cosmetic procedures available and other strategies that may be beneficial.[7] For example, facial fillers (such as Sculptra® or other implants) mask the appearance of lipoatrophy (fat loss) in the face. This procedure does not cure lipoatrophy and may need to be repeated. For lipohypertrophy (excess fat accumulation), liposuction can remove the unwanted fat pads ("buffalo hump" behind the neck). Some clinicians switch medications to try to slow or stop lipodystrophy. For example, switching your HIV drugs away from zidovudine (AZT, Retrovir®) and stavudine (d4T, Zerit®) may help slow lipoatrophy (fat loss) and possibly, with enough time, partially reverse it. Again, a switch strategy will depend on your prior treatment experience. Consult your doctor to see which of these strategies is right for you.

Keep Your Mind Active

The MacArthur Studies of Successful Aging found that people who are better educated, are physically active, have good lung function, and have high self-efficacy are most likely to maintain sharper mental ability.[8] To improve cognitive functioning they recommend memory training, involvement in social support, and increasing self-efficacy (the belief that one can deal with their problems appropriately).

Strategies recommended to maintain and increase cognitive functioning in middle-aged and older people living with HIV include reducing alcohol and substance use, improving nutrition, diminishing the effects of comorbidities, increasing social contact, reducing depression and stress levels, engaging in cognitively stimulating activities, applying cognitive remediation therapies, and incorporating psychopharmacological intervention.[9] Research in this area is at a nascent stage. If you are concerned about memory loss, talk to your doctor to develop a treatment plan tailored for your needs.

Develop a Health Care Regimen

Health care rituals involve taking your medications at the same time every day, eating meals at regular times, making time for exercise and relaxation, posting appointments on an easily accessible calendar, and so forth. These rituals are not meant to create rigidity in your life, but to help you prioritize and remember your health care. Performing daily rituals can help you feel more in control of your health and improve the way you feel both physically and emotionally.

Stop Smoking

Probably one of the single most important things you can do to improve your health is to stop smoking. The damaging effects of cigarette smoke, such as emphysema and lung cancer, to name two, are well documented. There is evidence that the harmful effects are even greater in people living with HIV, making smoking cessation more important.[10] There are numerous smoking cessation programs available. Contact your local health department. Your doctor has tools and medications to help you quit, too, such as nicotine replacement (gums, patches) as well as medications such as wellbutrin (Zyban®) and varenicline (Chantix®).

Reduce Drugs and Alcohol

The damaging effects of alcohol and drug abuse for people living with HIV and in the general aging population cannot be stressed enough. For example, "crystal meth" (methamphetamine) can lead to faster progression of HIV disease. Cocaine is associated with heart disease (including heart attack) and alters immune system function (including T cells). With increasing evidence that HIV itself may contribute to heart disease, it is important to lower your risk.

As for alcohol, although "two drinks per day" (a drink being 12 ounces of beer, 8 ounces of malt liquor, 5 ounces of wine, 1.5 ounces or "a shot" of 80-proof liquor) is considered "moderate drinking," there is no medical evidence that this is a safe amount in HIV-infected men. For men in the general population, drinking more than two drinks per day or more than four in one sitting indicates excessive drinking. The harmful effects of excessive drinking are well known (increased accidents, chronic diseases such as liver disease, pancreatitis, alcoholism). In HIV, excessive drinking is associated with increased medical and psychiatric complications, lower adherence to HIV medications, and poorer outcomes.

If drinking or drug use is interfering in your relationships, your social commitments (family, work, or school), or how you think or feel, you may have a drinking problem. The AA website, www .aa.org, has a list of questions you can ask yourself if you think alcohol or drugs are a problem for you. Talk to your doctor about your alcohol consumption and any drug use.

Maintain a Healthy Diet

When we age we lose muscle mass and require fewer calories daily. Uncontrolled HIV can accelerate the loss of muscle mass. If you are concerned about HIV wasting you may be tempted to overeat. Without adequate exercise, this may result in excess fat which raises the risk of developing (or worsening) other chronic conditions such as diabetes and heart disease. This is why nutrition and exercise are so important to help you maintain your muscle mass. Nutrition is particularly important if you have other medical problems (such as high blood pressure, high cholesterol, diabetes, or prediabetes) or lipodystrophy. A balanced diet is important to help your body fight HIV and control (or prevent) those other conditions.

A good place to start is to assess your overall dietary habits. In general, you want to eat a balanced diet with plenty of fresh fruits and vegetables. A good rule of thumb is called the "plate method." This is a simple way to devise a healthy meal and is recommended by the American Diabetes Association. Take your dinner plate and divide it in half. Fill one half with nonstarchy vegetables (such as spinach, broccoli, cauliflower, greens, salad, tomato, cucumber). Divide the remaining half again into two quarters. Fill one quarter with starchy foods (such as rice, pasta, corn, peas, whole grain breads/cereals). Fill the remaining quarter with proteins (lean meats, skinless poultry, seafood, tofu, eggs). Add a glass of nonfat or 1% milk or yogurt and a piece of fresh fruit. You can bring the plate method to the breakfast, lunch, or dinner table.

Consider the following small modifications. If you eat too much, try to limit your portions. If you drink soda, switch to seltzer or diet sodas. Avoid fast food. Switch to healthy oils, such as, olive oil or canola oil, and avoid food with trans fats.

Depending on your situation, your nutritional needs may differ. For example, if you are fighting an opportunistic infection, your calorie requirements may be higher than usual. If you have heart disease, diabetes, or other complications, you may have specific dietary restrictions. Ask about nutrition. You may also want to consult with a nutritionist to assess your dietary needs. Referrals for finding a good nutritionist and diet recommendations for aging and living with HIV are included as resources below.

Exercise Regularly

A balance of aerobic excercise, strength training, and stretching helps cardiovascular health while maintaining muscle mass, balance, and flexibility. There is evidence that physical exercise can actually forestall the onset of non-HIV-related dementia.[11] Aerobic activity gets your heart rate up. Calisthenics, rapid walking, jogging, dancing, and hiking are aerobic activities. Strength training—using weights or other forms of resistance—is increasingly found to be important for building muscle mass lost with aging. Weight machines, free weights, resistance bands, and exercise classes such as Pilates are all forms of strength training. Stretching is an important part of any exercise, especially to increase flexibility as we age. Yoga is an ancient form of exercise involving the mastery of postures that increase flexibility and strength. Exercise does not need to be strenuous. Start slowly with achievable goals and know your limits. You may want to consider getting started with a fitness professional. Before starting an exercise program be sure to discuss it with your doctor.

Get Enough Rest

Sleep disorders are common, but they don't have to be tolerated. Having trouble falling asleep or staying asleep can be signs of stress, depression, or anxiety. However, many people's sleep habits interfere with getting a good night's sleep. For example, eating or drinking in bed, reading or playing cards in bed, and falling asleep with the TV on for background noise are just a few. These practices train your body to be awake in bed. If you are having sleep problems, try retraining yourself: go to sleep and get up at the same time every day, remove the TV from the bedroom, make your bedroom quiet and dark (use blackout shades if necessary), do not read in bed, and do not eat or drink in bed. The bed should be only for sleep (and sex). Establish a prebedtime ritual, such as turning off the TV and computer at least 30–60 minutes before bedtime, changing out of your day clothes, and flossing and brushing your teeth, to prepare your body for sleep. When you feel tired, go to bed. If you cannot sleep after 20 minutes, get up and leave the bedroom, but don't turn on the TV or computer. Wait until you feel tired and try again. Recommended reading to help with sleep training is included in the resources section. If you continue to have trouble sleeping, you should bring it up with your doctor.

Take Your Vitamins and Minerals

Your needs for vitamins and minerals change as you age with HIV. Calcium supplements (with vitamin D) and multivitamins are recommended in the general elderly population. Folic acid and Vitamins B_6, B_{12}, and C are frequently prescribed as well. For people living with HIV, there is evidence of vitamin deficiencies, such as vitamins A and D. These deficiencies are usually managed with a healthy diet and multivitamin supplement.

There is a market for mega-vitamins and supplements to manage illnesses and aging. Be careful. It is possible to overdose on vitamins and minerals, causing toxic effects.

Other dietary supplements, such as fish oils, may be appropriate, particularly if you have high triglycerides (a type of fat). Some people like to take herbal preparations as well. Know that some herbal treatments (such as St. John's Wort and garlic supplements) can interact with your medications. Herbal supplements are generally unregulated by the FDA and there are no standards for purity. A note about side effects: many people believe that because herbal supplements are natural they have no side effects. This is not true. Everything has the potential for side effects. Talk to your doctor before starting or adding any supplement to your daily regimen.

Touch and Be Touched

Physical touch is an important part of physical health. Even if you are celibate, professional massages or hugs from friends can provide the healing powers of touch. Unsafe sex, however, undermines your physical health by putting your health at risk and may undermine your self-esteem. Review the chapter on sex in Section I where we discuss healthy sexuality and sexual function. Just as you should reexamine your exercise routine regularly to see if it's still working for you, you should reevaluate your sex life to see if your needs are being met.

Obstacles to Caring for Your Physical Health

There is a great deal of information covered in this section, and it only covers the basics of developing a healthy regimen of self-care. It is easy to become overwhelmed when managing the physical changes of aging with HIV. Some common obstacles you may encounter as you tackle the complex job of self-care are:

"It's too much." Take each section one at a time. When the information feels overwhelming put it aside and return to it later.

"This does not pertain to me." Do not skip any one recommendation. Be careful of rationalizations that downplay the importance of diet, drinking, or other topics. It is likely that the one area that you want to avoid is the most challenging to you.

"I've had HIV for a long time and know how to take care of myself." Our aging bodies are always changing and what once worked may not be the best self-care strategy as we get older.

"This information is out of date." Yes, it very well may be. It is your job to keep abreast of recent developments in the fields of aging and HIV.

Taking care of your physical health can sometimes feel like a full-time job, and you may want a vacation. Remember, self-care is an act of self-love. You deserve the best that you can offer.

Resources

The Gay Men's Health Crisis' website, www.gmhc.org, offers information on finding a doctor and entering clinical trials.

The AA website, www.aa.org, has a list of questions you can ask yourself if you think alcohol or drugs are a problem for you.

AIDS Project Los Angeles has a comprehensive list of recommendations and articles about nutrition and HIV at www.apla .org/programs/nutrition.html. *Healthy Aging: A Lifelong Guide to Your Well-Being*, by Andrew Weil, M.D., offers a nutrition plan for optimum aging.

See www.thebody.com/index/treat/herbal.html for detailed information and links on diet and nutrition. The American Diabetes Association has suggestions about diabetes and the plate method on their website, www.diabetes.org.

For information about yoga and HIV, go to www.yogagroup.org.

A good book to help you develop good sleep habits is *Learn to Sleep Well: A Practical Guide to Getting a Good Night's Rest*, by Chris Idzikowski.

Step 2

Rebuild and Maintain Your Social Networks

Why Rebuild Your Social Network?

At this point I hope you see that having a rich social support system is integral to optimal aging with HIV. In Chapter 3 we reviewed some of the science on social support. We identified how having friends and family mitigates the challenges of living with HIV and of aging in general. We demonstrated that the presence or absence of social support affects your physical health and emotional well-being. We also pointed out that it is not merely the number of friends that is important, but your satisfaction with those supports that matters. In that chapter we also showed how your needs for, interest in, and access to support from friends have changed over the years.

In Chapter 4 we examined the significant role the gay community once provided as a form of social support, noting that you may rely less on the community today. And in Chapter 7 we discussed how your role in the family has changed, and we helped you to determine whether family can provide support to you as you age with HIV. Finally, in Chapter 11 we demonstrated how the combination of loss, illness, and changing priorities has constricted your circles of social involvement and how living within limitations can create a shrinking kind of life.

Step 2 will offer you some basic tools to rebuild your social networks and make sure that you are getting the support you need to enter the next phase of your life with the foundation necessary to meet the challenges ahead. To accomplish this, I will lead you through three basic questions: *What* do you need friends for? *Who* do you want to add to your life? And *how* can you find them?

What Do You Need Friends for?

Before you can take steps to rebuild your social network, you must first determine what you need in a friend. In Chapter 3 you completed an exercise in which you formed a self-care corporation. Through that exercise you identified your needs for emotional, instrumental, and informational support.

Your emotional support is made up of friends who are there for you with all of your feelings—whether you are sad, angry, hurt, disappointed, happy, exhilarated, or bored. Your instrumental support system provides assistance in accomplishing tasks, such as taking you to the doctor, doing chores around the house, or providing a meal when you are ill. You receive informational support from an expert/friend, such as someone who knows the entitlement system or who is well versed in HIV medications and their side effects.

Defining what you need in a friend is integral to rebuilding satisfying support networks. You may have a number of older friends on whose shoulders you can cry but no one who can reach that jar of pickles on the top shelf. Conversely, you may have many acquaintances who are willing to help out if you are in a jam, but who aren't intimate enough to talk with about your feelings. As you review your self-care exercise consider what positions remain unfilled.

Who Do You Need as a Friend?

Here, too, you need to do some preliminary work to ensure that there is a "goodness of fit" between your needs and what your friends can offer. First, consider what works best for you. When you are down, do you feel most comfortable sitting at home with a quiet friend, or do you need someone to get you out of your shell? Do you like it when people check in with you regularly on the phone, or does that feel too intrusive? Would you prefer to have a standing date for coffee, or to get together spontaneously? Next, evaluate your friends' strengths and weaknesses. Do you have a great friend whose shoulder you can always cry on, but she's really no fun to be around when you're in a playful mood? Or do you have someone for whom you care deeply, but he just doesn't "get it" when you are anxious? When you look for a friend to fill those empty positions make sure that you are selecting someone who has the ability to meet your needs.

How Do You Rebuild Your Social Network?

Determining *how* you can fill those positions is a two-step process. First, you must consider whether you are adequately using your existing networks. Do you have friendships that can be deepened? You may have people in your life who would welcome the chance to become better friends if given the chance. Relationships grow with greater intimacy. You can move that process along by spending more time with your friends, sharing personal stories, telling your friends how much they matter to you, showing up for them in a supportive way, letting them know more about your personal feelings, confiding in them, and asking for help when you need it.

The second way to build your support network is to look for people on whom you think you can rely. That can feel risky, but it is imperative for your well-being that you take the chance. Of course, emotionally supportive relationships tend to develop over time and you can't always know whether someone will be a good friend when you first get to meet them. Here, environment is important. It's more likely you will find someone interested in building an intimate relationship at a social service organization helping the bereaved than at a website frequented by young men looking for casual sex. This point may seem obvious, but in my practice in psychotherapy I have heard many stories of men getting rejected by people they thought they connected with. Only later, in hindsight, do my clients see that the person was clearly interested only in sex when they met. One way to improve the chances of meeting a like-minded soul is to seek out friends at clubs or agencies for people with shared interests and concerns.

Consider rebuilding your social network at the HIV, gay, spiritual, and other community-based organizations in your area.

Another avenue to finding greater intimacy in your life is to join a support group. HIV support groups were once a rite of passage for gay men living with HIV. You may benefit from being in a group of people who share your experience and who you can expect will "get it" when you talk about your past, your current concerns, and your feelings. Support groups provide opportunities for mutual aid, understanding, a universalizing experience, and personal growth. And you may make friendships that extend beyond the life of the group. In many self-help groups you are advised to try six meetings before you determine whether a group is right for you. The resources section will offer some suggestions concerning organizations to contact in your effort to find a group.

You should also consider psychotherapy. A professional psycho-therapist can provide emotional support and help you work through the obstacles that stand in the way of forming more inti-mate relationships. One way to find a therapist is by word of mouth. Ask people you know who they would recommend, or contact your doctor, local gay community center, or HIV service organization for a referral. You can also get a great deal of informa-tion about a psychotherapist on the Internet. Some websites on which you can start a search are listed as resources.

Here are a few suggestions for rebuilding your social network:

- *Renew old acquaintances.* Contact friends from your past or deepen your involvement with extended family.
- *Seek out people with whom you have things in common.* Join an organization. Many of the men I spoke with are in HIV or gay men's support groups. But the options are as broad as your interests. Are you into doll collecting? Environmental issues? Chess? *The Avengers?* Macrobiotic cooking? Salsa dancing? There is a club for you. Look at your local gay community organization, AIDS service agency, newspaper, or on the web to find a group that fits your needs.
- *Talk to a stranger.* Strike up a conversation with someone you see at the supermarket, in the building where you live, or the restaurant on the corner. If you don't know what to say, ask a question. People love to talk about themselves

- *Diversify your networks.* Your friends should include people from different backgrounds. The wider and more varied your network, the greater your ability to manage what life throws at you. There may be straight, younger, or HIV-negative people in your life who would welcome the opportunity to develop a closer bond.
- *Don't wait for people to contact you.* If you want to talk to someone, pick up the phone (and leave a message at the beep). Every day. I don't know anyone who can read minds. No one will know that you need help if you don't ask for it.
- *Consider professional supports.* You may feel more comfortable reaching out to a psychotherapist, pastoral counselor, or social worker than a friend when you are depressed or anxious.
- *Get a pet.* Pets are great companions. And when you're walking the dog, who knows who you might meet?
- *Pursue (or maintain) a romantic relationship.* A stable marriage at age 50 is one of the predictors of healthy aging at age 75.[1]
- *Use the Internet to cast a wider net.* The Internet is not a replacement for human contact, but it can be an effective tool to rebuild your social network. Several organizations on aging serving the lesbian, gay, bisexual, and transgender (LGBT) and HIV communities have resources on the web. Don't be afraid to join Facebook, Twitter, or LinkedIn. They are great tools to stay in touch with people of all ages.
- *Form a reading group.* At the end of the book I outline a strategy to use this book in a group setting. But you can form a reading group on any subject that interests you. Start advertising by word of mouth and then consider where you can post a flier or put in an ad to best reach like-minded people, such as your office or a local bookstore.

Maintaining Social Networks

Building and rebuilding social networks are useful only if you keep those relationships active. Friendships don't form overnight. Just as a garden needs constant tending before your new plant can take root, you must nurture your relationships for them to mature. Keep showing up. Stay in regular contact with your friends. Time and distance can weaken the bonds of friendship. Find ways to stay in touch, such as the telephone or Internet. Similarly, don't allow arguments or miscommunication to jeopardize a good friendship. Try to work out your disagreements by talking to each other, or ask a friend or professional counselor to help you mediate the problem. Remember, maintaining friendships is as important as forming them.

Obstacles to Rebuilding Social Networks

If I had a quarter for every time I heard the following story, I would be a millionaire: A client tells me that he was feeling ill and called an ambulance. After sitting alone in the emergency room for hours, he is seen by a doctor who says that there is noth-ing she can do and he is referred back to his internist. The client then takes a taxi home.

When he sees his doctor next, he describes the incident, only to be asked, "Why didn't you call my office first?" When he sees his friends, they ask, "Why didn't you call me? I would have gone to the doctor with you." "I would have sat with you in the ER." "I would have given you a ride home."

The primary obstacle to rebuilding your social network is inter-nal. And in order to regain your path to optimal aging with HIV you must first ask yourself why you don't reach out to others. Here are some common obstacles to asking for help:

"There is no one available." You may feel that age and illness have reduced your social network to nothing and that there is no one left for you. But as the above scenario demonstrates, there is always someone to whom you can turn for help, even if you don't yet know him or her.

"I don't want to be a burden." One common misconception is that when we feel overwhelmed by our problems we think that other people will feel that way too. My years as a volunteer coor-dinator have taught me that it is actually easier to listen to some-one else, give advice, and offer assistance with other people's problems than it is to solve our own. People who volunteer their

time to help others often express gratitude that they get far more out of the experience than they give.

"I don't need any help." Man is a social animal. When we are too self-sufficient we limit our opportunities for life-enhancing contact with others. Being vulnerable is part of the human condition. Recognizing your needs is acknowledging your humanity.

"I'm afraid of rejection." Yes, it is true that rejection is painful. But when we experience pain and work through it we have opportunities for growth. Consider whether the pain of rejection is truly more than you can take and if it is really worth the suffering you experience from isolating yourself.

"I'm too shy." Some people are more outgoing than others, but if your shyness is getting in the way of your making friends you may have low self-esteem or social anxiety. Consider counseling or joining a group to overcome insecurity in social situations.

"I'm too tired." It may seem exhausting to contemplate reaching out to others when you are ill. But research on aging and chronicity has taught us that the more you do, the more you can do. Conversely, illness can lead to a downward spiral of isolation, depression, and physical deterioration. If you feel too ill to go out, make sure you have regular visits with friends and family, or contact a local social service organization for a visiting volunteer.

"I don't want to experience any more loss." Every time we enter into a relationship we risk loss. When you reach out to others you take the chance that they may leave you. And recognizing the need for new friends means acknowledging the space created by old losses. To withstand the losses inherent in life we must be resilient in our ability to grieve. In Step 5 we will examine the process of grief and help you remove this obstacle to rebuilding your life.

"I'm too depressed." Withdrawal, apathy toward life, lack of motivation, reduced interest in people, and fatigue can all be symptoms of depression. When you are depressed the idea of rebuilding your social network seems overwhelming. But depression is treatable and part of the strategy of overcoming depression is to break the concomitant patterns of isolation. If you believe that you might be suffering from depression there are tools available to help you. We will review them in more depth in Step 6.

It takes work to rebuild and maintain a support network, but having people to rely on as you age with HIV is well worth the effort.

Resources

Services and Advocacy for GLBT Elders (SAGE) (online at www.sageusa.org) has services for the LBGT and HIV-positive communities.

The Senior HIV Intervention Project (SHIP) (online at www .browardchd.org/services/AIDS/ship.htm), is a health program in Broward County, Florida, that specifically addresses the needs of people over 50 with HIV.

Gay Men's Health Crisis (GMHC), in New York (online at www.gmhc.org), and Openhouse, in San Francisco, (online at openhouse-sf.org), offer services to middle-aged and older people living with HIV. They may also be able to direct you to programs in your area.

New York Association on HIV Over Fifty (NYAHOF) (online at www.nyahof.org) is a clearinghouse of information and resources for people throughout the nation.

American Society of Aging LGBT Aging Resources Clearing-house (online at www.asaging.org/larc) offers information on services in the LGBT communities nationwide.

AARP has a comprehensive website (www.aarp.org) with articles, information, and referrals throughout the country on a wide range of topics of interest to middle-aged and older people.

Step 3

Be Generative

What Is Generativity?

In Chapter 9 we defined the challenge of generativity vs. stagnation. At midlife we can either be generative through procreation, production, and creativity, passing on our knowledge to others, or we can stagnate in self-absorption, shrinking away from youth, productivity, and the concerns of others. Eric Erikson, who developed the eight-stage model for understanding human development, believed that in middle age, "mature man needs to be needed"[1] and that generativity is integral to continued development through midlife and beyond. Although this life stage model has been criticized for being too normative, culminating in the expression of middle class values, and inconsiderate of diversity in class, race, ethnicity, as well as sexual orientation,[2] the concept of generativity has been reconsidered, reshaped, and applied to the field of gay aging.[3]

For gay men aging with HIV, generativity can play a significant role in rebuilding social networks and reclaiming lives given up to the virus. In Chapter 8 you explored how career, once a central feature of life, has shifted in importance over the years. You identified the positive aspects of work, including making money, having a social outlet, involvement in creative pursuits, competition, and building self-esteem. You considered whether your current involvement in generative activities through work and volunteering offers you opportunities to receive those benefits today.

Why You Should Be Generative

Section II explored the real threat that stagnation poses for gay men aging with HIV. Through an exploration of the literature we demonstrated that stagnation at midlife can lead to self-absorption, feeling little connection to others, isolation, and a lack of any sense of meaning in life. I asked four questions to help you identify where you might be stuck, and using the men's stories as evidence, I demonstrated how stagnation can lead to isolation, living in the past, accepting the status quo, and avoiding the future.

In Chapter 12 we demonstrated through the research the positive effects generativity can have on physical and emotional well-being as we age. You examined how being involved in generative pursuits can combat the tendency to get stuck in your ways at midlife. And you saw that generativity counteracts stagnation through the act of giving of oneself to the next generation.

The benefits of generativity are numerous. Being involved in activities to care for others involves you in a community outside yourself and helps you remain socially integrated at midlife. Generativity also solves the problem of finding creativity, play, and competition in work and retirement. And by being involved in the life of someone younger you can visit youth without living in the past.

Generativity reminds you of what you have to offer. Age and experience have won you hard-earned wisdom. But what good is your knowledge if you don't share it with others? Through mentoring or acting as a coach, leader, or consultant, you remind yourself of the skills you have to offer.

Finally, generative activities offer you opportunities for personal growth. When we teach others, we learn about ourselves. The unexpected challenges of working with others give us important information about ourselves and keep us on our toes, pushing ourselves to grow with the people we are helping.

How You Can Be Generative

You can be generative through involvement with children, mentoring young adults, volunteering to assist and educate others, acting as a consultant, guide, and coach, or any activity that keeps you participating in the larger society, caring for others, and passing on your wisdom.

Here are a few ideas about how you can add generativity to your life:

- Take on a supervisory position at work
- Teach a class or workshop
- Lead a social group
- Tutor a child
- Provide companionship to a homebound person
- Become politically active
- Be an HIV peer educator
- Serve on a community advisory board
- Mentor gay teens
- Join a professional organization
- Start an advice column or blog
- Write a self-help book

Obstacles to Generativity

Many of the obstacles to participating in generative activities are the same as those that interfere with any social involvement. Being too shy and afraid of rejection, fatigue, fear of personal involvement and future losses, and depression can all impede your ability to put yourself out there to help others. There are some additional rationalizations I have heard in my work that are given as reasons to avoid generative pursuits.

"I have enough troubles taking care of myself." It may be true that you are burdened by caring for yourself. However, helping others is rewarding, and my work with volunteers has taught me that the energy spent on caring for someone else is usually returned with interest. As an additional benefit, being involved in generative activity provides a break from your own troubles by getting you out of yourself and immersed in someone else's life.

"I have nothing to offer." Your life's experience has given you wisdom, strength, and skills necessary to guide a younger person through his or her own personal growth. But you need to appreciate what you have to offer in order to help someone else. We can

all feel insecure at time, but if low self-esteem makes you feel as though you have nothing to offer you may want to consider psychotherapy to help you build your self-confidence.

Get involved. It's not too late for you to pursue your goals, to find new interests, or to have an impact on someone else for the better. You have a great deal to offer the world, but you are of no service to anyone, including yourself, if you don't put yourself out there.

Resources

The LBGT community center in New York has volunteer opportunities, or contact your local gay center at www.gaycenter.org.

Volunteer to work with gay kids at Hetrick-Martin Institute, in New York (online at www.hmi.org).

AARP can help you find local volunteer opportunities (online at www.createthegood.org).

Step 4

Fight the Triple Threat: AIDS Stigma, Homophobia, and Ageism

What Is the Triple Threat?

The literature on HIV over 50 often refers to the "triple threat" gay men face as they age with HIV.[1] You have had to face the stigma of homophobia, AIDS, and, now, ageism and together they can create obstacles to your optimal aging with HIV.

Let's first define each stigma and discuss its impact on your history and life today.

Homophobia

We reviewed your history facing the homophobia of your youth in Chapter 4 and helped you remember its impact on your physical and emotional health, and in Chapter 7 you recalled how growing up gay impacted your family history. In Chapter 4 you remembered both the trauma and the liberation of coming out and identified the important role the gay community had in combating the effects of homophobia and rebuilding your self-esteem.

You recognized that although there have been changes in society, homophobia still exists. And we examined some of the research on homophobia in the form of institutionalized oppression (in the law, housing, employment, marriage, and health care, among others), the real threat of physical violence, emotional abuse and verbal assault, and stereotyping in the media and how it creates an environment of stigma. Homophobia can be subtle and insidious, or blatant and life-threatening. Identifying where the threat of homophobia exists in your life can be a challenge in and of itself.

In Chapter 4 we examined how a lifetime of homophobia can be internalized, affecting the way you relate to yourself and others. It is almost impossible to live through the pervasive antigay messages in this culture and not be affected. Even after years of self-love and acceptance we see the residual effects of internalized homophobia expressed in guilt about sex, shame about our sexual orientation, distancing ourselves from others, intimacy issues, and insecurity about our self-worth. The relationship between internalized homophobia and depression, alcohol abuse, high-risk behaviors, and low self-esteem has been documented in the literature.[2] Combating internalized homophobia involves a lifelong process of looking inward to consider how gay oppression has shaped our view of ourselves.

AIDS Stigma

AIDS is a stigmatized illness. There was a time, not long ago, when people were refused treatment in hospitals. Today, the stigma against HIV disease is still present, and people living with the virus are made to feel unsafe and unwelcome in health care settings, social service organizations, communities, religious groups, workplaces, and families. As we discussed in Chapter 2, people living with lipodystrophy often feel that they carry the "look of AIDS" and that it affects the way friends, family, and strangers interact with them. Whenever you feel like you are treated differently because of your HIV status, you are experiencing the sting of AIDS stigma.

Ageism

In Chapter 4 you identified the realities of ageism in the gay community and in the world at large. And in Chapter 8 you recognized that although discriminating on the base of age in the workplace is illegal, you face subtle (and sometimes not so subtle) forms of age-related stigma at work and other areas of your life. If you feel invisible, less valuable, weak, or unwelcome because of your age, that is ageism. In Chapter 9 you saw how recognizing your aging contributes to your continued psychological and emotional development. And you identified the ageist attitudes that you may be harboring, including beliefs that older people are "past it," less interesting, unattractive, or frail.

Other Stigmas

Of course, there are many other stigmas in this country. Discrimination based on race, ethnicity, religious background, sex, gender identity/gender expression, psychiatric diagnosis, or physical ability is a real concern that you may be facing in your life. As we discussed in Chapter 4, it is integral that you find people who understand your experience in order to help you manage the stigma of being different. The resources section includes some organizations you can contact for support.

Why Is It Imperative That You Confront the Triple Stigma?

Combating the effects of stigma is integral to optimal aging with HIV. When you do not remain adaptive to the changes associated with aging, you can become stagnant in middle age. Stigma affects your ability to adapt by limiting your options, creating rigidity in your coping strategies, and reducing your social involvement. Ageism can also impact your approach to growing older. As Dr. Andrew Weil explains, "If aging is written into the laws of the universe, then acceptance of it must be a prerequisite for doing it in a graceful way."[3] In Chapter 9 you identified some of your own attitudes about aging. You saw how negative beliefs about older people can lead you to think less of yourself, affect your social involvement, and impact your belief that age has offered you strengths, wisdom, and abilities to do whatever a younger person can. Ageist attitudes are deeply ingrained in our society, and we may have internalized them without our conscious awareness. The strategies used to combat both external and internal ageism are similar to those you may have developed to fight homophobia and AIDS stigma.

How to Fight the Triple Stigma

Fighting the triple threat means confronting the realities of homophobia, AIDS stigma, and ageism in your external and internal worlds. Through my years of experience running workshops, providing individual therapy, and facilitating groups I have come to appreciate the complexities of this challenge. It is a lifelong task to determine whether threats of abuse are real or imagined, past or present. And deciding the best way to take care of ourselves when we feel the sting of stigma involves the ability to assess a situation, the people involved, and our abilities at that moment. I will approach the complexities of this topic from the outside in, by examining how to address overt forms of discrimination as well as more subtle forms, and finally by examining the ways in which we combat internalized stigma.

First you must identify where the realities of stigma exist in your present life. Consider areas in which you may be living with overt forms of homophobia, AIDS stigma, and ageism and decide the safest course you can take to protect yourself. Fighting the triple stigma means not accepting mistreatment because you are gay, HIV positive, or older.

Verbal harassment from a stranger, friend, lover, or family member is abuse and should be treated as such. Protecting yourself by telling someone and seeking assistance when you feel you are the victim of physical assault or verbal harassment is one of the most significant ways you can fight the triple threat of stigma in your life. Physical assault because of your sexual orientation, HIV status, or age is a crime and should be reported to the police no matter who the perpetrator is. You can also contact an appropriate community-based organization to make sure that you are receiving the support you need. Victim service agencies are listed as resources below.

Facing stigma in your current life is often more than identifying and combating overt abuse. The triple threat of homophobia, AIDS stigma, and ageism can come in the form of discrimination. When we combat discriminatory policies in the legal system, in schools, in health care, in the media, and in other institutions we send an important message to ourselves and to others that gay, HIV-positive, and older people are valuable members of society entitled to equal treatment. By becoming involved in organizations that fight discrimination, writing letters, or speaking out we combat the triple threat of stigma and build our self-esteem.

Sometimes stigma can be more difficult to detect. It can be hard to determine whether you are being rejected in social situations, ignored by professionals, or discriminated against at work because of your sexual orientation, HIV status, or age. But you know when you feel uncomfortable. Trust that feeling. Can you say something to the person directly? Often people are unaware that their remarks or behavior can be perceived as insulting. Sometimes you can misunderstand a person's words or intentions. Talking it out gives you the opportunity to make your feelings known, stand up for yourself, clear up a miscommunication, or educate an ignorant person. If you don't feel safe saying something in the moment, talk it over with a friend. In either case, it is best for your emotional health that you process the experience with someone else so that you do not carry the stigma with you in the form of shame, resentment, and anger. When it comes to feeling stigmatized a good rule of thumb to remember is that if you didn't feel right, something wrong was going on.

The second way to fight the triple threat of stigma is to recognize how stigma from your past can be affecting your life today. No matter how subtle, or how long ago, abuse, rejection, discrimination, and oppression can leave invisible scars. One way we react to past wounds is to anticipate future threats. Sometimes our sensitivity is spot on and we can avoid situations that would make us unsafe or uncomfortable. But at other times, our anticipation of abuse and discrimination causes us to shy away from experiences when no threat is present. It takes rigorous honesty to recognize whether your fears are justified in the present or if they are rooted in experiences from your past. Consider where you may be shying away from social situations because you think you may be rejected because of your age, avoiding making new friends in your building for fear they may find out that you are gay, taking on new challenges at work because you imagine the straight guys will tease or alienate you, and avoiding contact with extended family for fear that they might shun you because of your HIV status. Whenever we try something new, there is always risk involved, but if your anticipation of stigma is based on your history of discrimination then you are only holding yourself back.

You must also recognize when the internalization of stigma may be expressing itself in your relationships with yourself and others. A lifetime of homophobia can result in negative self-esteem, shame, lack of intimacy, or self-destructive behavior. When we do not face our internalized homophobia, we can carry it with us, treating ourselves far worse than the people who abused us. Consider where your internalized homophobia may be hiding. Do you have low self-esteem? Are you self-critical? Are you embarrassed about your appearance? Negative attitudes toward yourself can all be expressions of internalized homophobia. What about your relationships with others? Do you have close gay friends? Do you judge other gay people harshly? Is it difficult to maintain intimate relationships? Often our internalized homophobia is expressed in the way we treat other gay people. Do you hurt yourself with alcohol or drugs? Is your spending out of control? Do you binge on food, or starve yourself? Is your sex life affirming or does it endanger your physical, emotional, or spiritual health? Compulsive and destructive behaviors can also be expressions of internalized homophobia.

Combating the internalizations of stigma can be a lifelong process. The best way to fight and undo the damage of homophobia is to take good care of yourself. If any of the issues above are current concerns seek out the appropriate support or self-help group. You can also work on these issues with other gay men in a support group or with a trained psychotherapist. The resources section of this step as well as the step "check your baggage" will offer you tips on finding the right support for you.

Finally, you must face your internalized ageism. What did you think about men your age when you were 20? Were they "old queens," "dirty, old men," "decrepit," and "past it" or "wise," "mature," "seasoned," and "tough"? Now that you are older do you apply these attributes to yourself?

Write two lists, one of the advantages and one of the disadvantages of growing older. Now, ask a friend to make the same list. Discuss your answers. Which of your responses are the same? Which are different? Were you surprised about anything on their list? Consider how your attitudes about aging affect the ways in which you care for yourself. Do your feelings about getting older affect the ways in which you relate to other people your age, younger or older? Does your age affect the choices you make on how you socialize or spend your time? Ask another person to make the list. Keep talking.

Obstacles to Addressing Stigma

Two common reactions to experiencing stigma are opposite sides of the same coin. We either downplay the importance of the event or we become overwhelmed by it. In either case, we do nothing. It is important to remember that in the aftermath of stigma, both are normal, but potentially damaging results. Stigma makes us feel that it is our fault, that we are responsible, deserving, or overly sensitive to negative attention because of our personal qualities. When we do not get support from others, we take the risk of isolating ourselves and allowing the stigma to negatively impact our self-esteem. I have heard people express internalized stigma in the following ways.

"It's not really that important." Reaction is different from overreaction. If you feel something is amiss, that means you are sensitive, not overly sensitive. You have a right to have those feelings validated.

"I'm afraid." Sometimes there is a risk to confront your abuser. If you are afraid to combat any form of oppression, seek out guidance from a professional with experience dealing with stigma.

"It happened so long ago, it no longer affects me." Sometimes time heals all wounds. Sometimes those wounds just fester. Unfortunately, stigma can have long-lasting and subtle affects. If you find that the stigma of your past is negatively affecting your self-esteem or social interaction talk to someone else.

Some theorists believe that gay people are well equipped to manage the challenges of aging and, that by surviving the coming out experience and gay oppression we have developed a "crisis competence" that gives us a perspective on major life challenges and provides a buffer from the vicissitudes of aging.[4] When you confront the internal and external effects of stigma you remove significant obstacles to optimal aging with HIV.

Resources

Organizations such as the Gay and Lesbian Anti-Violence Project (AVP) and the Gay and Lesbian Alliance Against Defamation (GLAAD) can help you figure out the best way to handle discrimination. Local gay organizations can help you face the effects of homophobia in your life. To find a local organization contact www.gaycenter.org or the Audre Lorde Project at www .ALP.org, which has an extensive resource list of LGBT and HIV organizations serving the diverse communities of people of color in New York and may help you find a group in your area.

Two good books can help you address internalized homophobia: *Golden Men: The Power of Gay Midlife*, by Harold Kooden and *Loving Ourselves: The Gay and Lesbian Guide to Self-Esteem*, by Dr. Kimeron Hardin.

Healthy Aging: A Lifelong Guide to Your Well-Being by Dr. Andrew Weil has tips for dealing with ageism in yourself and others. Also see *Stigma: Notes on the Management of Spoiled Identity*, by Erving Goffman.

Step 5

Let Yourself Grieve

Why Grieving Is Important

I believe that one of the greatest threats to optimal aging with HIV is unresolved grief. I have met many gay men who are so overwhelmed with the sadness, anger, powerlessness, and guilt of multiple losses that they are unable to live on and make the most of their lives. Sometimes they are unaware of the depth of these feelings. But their behavior demonstrates that they are stuck in mourning. Two signs of stagnation—living in the past and leading a shrinking kind of life—are both, coincidentally, symptoms of unresolved grief.

Letting yourself grieve means acknowledging and feeling the loss without becoming consumed by it. I am not advocating that you become mired in the sadness of lost loves. Quite the contrary. I believe that in order to live in the present and build a future you must be able to mourn the past. When you allow yourself to grieve and feel all your feelings, you can let them pass. Feelings come and go. Sadness is just another feeling. When you let yourself feel sadness, and all the emotions of grief, in a safe and supportive environment, they, too, will eventually pass and allow for new feelings to emerge.

Neither does mourning the past mean moving on and forgetting about people, places, and activities that are no longer. Successful mourning allows you to have access to your past memories. In Chapter 10 we examined the healing power of reminiscence.

You saw how remembering the past can remind you of skills you once had, build on the good of past relationships, and draw from the love and guidance once offered by people no longer in your life. When you can let yourself grieve you are no longer afraid to remember past loves and you are free to let your memories support you in the present.

What Losses Are There to Grieve?

There are many kinds of losses. In fact, whenever you experience a change, even one for the better, there is a loss involved. As children when we go to school for the first time we have to say good-bye to life at home with our primary guardian. But experiencing that loss opens up the whole world to us.

Throughout the book we have identified the losses inherent to aging with HIV. In Chapter 1 you explored the losses created by the AIDS epidemic. You may not have lost many friends to AIDS. However, AIDS took a whole generation of gay men. Even if your personal losses were few, their death created a loss in the community as a whole. The AIDS epidemic ended a way of life, and mourning the losses of AIDS not only involves grieving the past but also the future you anticipated for yourself before the epidemic.

In Chapter 2 you saw how illness and age both create losses, and how in order to adapt to the physical and financial changes involved in each you have had to mourn the loss of what you once could do. In Chapters 3 through 7 you appreciated the significant gap created by loss of friends, lovers, and family members and saw how illness and death reshaped your role and identity. Not all losses involved death, and you considered how break-ups and other separations needed to be mourned in order to move on with your life. In Chapter 8 you saw how work itself could be seen as a relationship that needed to be mourned so that you could appreciate what you got out of it and look for ways to receive those benefits today. Finally, in Chapter 9 you saw how personal growth is a continual process of assessment, discarding, and rebuilding ways of viewing yourself and relating to others. Mourning loss is endemic to all these processes.

The most difficult loss to articulate is deeply internal. Part of the mourning process involves grieving what we never received, but hoped for. Sometimes this involves accepting the limitations of our parents and acknowledging that we did not receive all that we needed from them. Dreams, too, should be mourned. When we grieve our fantasies of what we wished our lives could have been we allow our experience and maturity to reshape our goals. Mourning the dreams of our youth allows us to say goodbye to what was never achieved in order to live more fully in the present.

Grieving your losses is an integral part of adapting to aging with HIV. When you cannot grieve you do not say goodbye. You remain either mired in the past or completely closed off to it. In either case unresolved grief can lead to stagnation in midlife, limiting your available resources in your attempt to adapt to aging with HIV.

How Do We Grieve?

In my work as a psychotherapist I am often called on to help people through the process of mourning. Initially, this work involves overcoming the initial shock and disbelief of loss. Helping someone take in the reality of a loss is an integral step in the grieving process. Avoidance strategies, such as numbness and denying emotions, need to be broken down as well. Although numbness may seem preferable to experiencing painful grief, it is counter productive to integrating loss in a healthy way. Mourners in this phase can fool others by appearing to accept the loss and appearing to take it well, when they are actually avoiding feelings of grief and postponing and complicating their mourning process.

The second phase of grief work involves working through the feelings of loss. There are no "right" feelings when it comes to grief and no correct order in which to feel your feelings. The common reactions to dying outlined by Dr. Elisabeth Kübler-Ross help us to understand the range of emotions we can experience in grief: denial, anger, bargaining, depression, and acceptance.[1] While some feelings may seem inappropriate, it is important to recognize that reactions to loss can be complex and powerful, and although they may not make sense at first, by allowing ourselves to have all of our feelings we can move through them more quickly into acceptance. For example, it is quite normal to be angry at the person who died. This is a way we express our frustration that someone we cared for is no longer with us. We may also feel guilty and be angry at ourselves because we believe we could have done something to prevent the person's death. Usually, this feeling is not based on fact, but is the way in which we react to the inevitability of mortality. Letting go of guilt is integral to managing feelings of powerlessness. These feelings can be quite intense at first and later come as waves with growing periods of calm between. Grief never comes to a complete end. We can always be stung, sometimes unexpectedly, by the pain of grief. Anniversaries, holidays, people, places, food, and even smells can trigger old grief. Every new loss has the potential to resurrect past mourning.

You can begin to resolve grief when you accept the loss, and when the feelings of loss no longer interfere with your daily life. Integrating loss means being able to return to old interests and activities. Memories are no longer accompanied by overwhelming sadness, and you can experience pleasure and fulfillment in your current life. Adapting to loss often involves rebuilding in a way that compensates for your loss. You will form new relationships, restructure your life, and develop skills to make up for the absence created through death.

Coping with loss is a personal journey. We manage the experience by drawing from a wealth of past experiences and individual strengths.[2] We recall how we managed deaths in our past to remind ourselves that we can survive the pain of grief. We can also draw on the experience of others, remembering, for example, how our friends and family dealt with death to gain strength and guidance. We should also turn to others for support. While solitary periods may be comforting, isolation at this time should be avoided. Mourning is rooted in culture. You may find yourself repeating traditions that you have not remembered in years. Connecting to history broadens our perspective on individual loss. As you let yourself grieve the losses that may be standing in the way of your optimal aging with HIV, consider the adaptive processes you've already developed.

Most cultures use ritual to assist in the grieving process. Funerals, wakes, and memorials all follow formal procedures to guide a mourner through the process of grief. Prayers, hymns, chanting, lighting candles, and eulogizing are all examples of rites to help us experience our sadness, to give and receive support, to honor the dead, to share warm memories and laughter, and to practice traditions that connect us to the past and to a power beyond ourselves. Prescribed rituals at anniversaries, such as visiting a grave or performing a service, give us opportunities to remember the loss and continue to process unresolved grief.

Find a ritual that works for you, such as a tradition from your family, religion, or community that was comforting in the past. Or you can create something new. Set aside a day or evening for a symbolic act that allows you to recognize your loss. Light a candle or look at old photos. Reflect on your grief. Let yourself have all your feelings. Write them down in a journal or tell someone else. You want to make sure you have enough support available from friends and family, that you are taking care of yourself with rest, healthy food, and adequate exercise, and that you are replenishing fluids by drinking plenty of water. You may need to repeat this act until you feel some sense of closure.

If you find that your feelings are becoming overwhelming, interfering with your functioning, affecting your appetite or sleep, or you are developing destructive patterns, such as drinking in excess or compulsive sex, you may be depressed. Talk about this with a friend or counselor. In the next step we will talk more about depression and give you tools for finding the right help.

Obstacles to Mourning

The following are some examples of complicated mourning.

"I have not experienced that much loss." No matter how great the loss, all losses affect us. Denying the significance of loss can be a maladaptive way of coping.

"I'm done with grief." Mourning is never over. Although the intense feelings of loss may be resolved, we can always be reminded of lost loves. When we are available to feelings of sadness they can pass freely.

"I don't like thinking about the past." Avoiding feelings of grief can prevent you from having access to positive memories.

"It's too upsetting for me." If thinking of people, places, and things from your past is too upsetting you may be suffering from depression; you should talk to your doctor or a mental health practitioner.

Letting yourself grieve is challenging work, but it is an integral step toward optimal aging with HIV. When you grieve you honor yourself and those that you lost and give yourself the psychic space to engage fully in your life today.

Resources

You can use the following books to help you through mourning:

The Other Side of Sadness: What the New Science of Bereavement Tells Us About Life After Loss by George Bonanno

On Death and Dying by Elisabeth Kubler-Ross

Healing After Loss: Daily Meditations for Working Through Grief by Martha Whitmore Hickman

The Tibetan Book on Living and Dying by Sogyal Rinpoche

Hospice of the North Shore has a website with information on the grief process: www.hns.org/Center_for_Grief_Healing/The _Grieving_Process.aspx.

The United States Department of Health website has referrals for grief counseling throughout the United States on their website: mentalhealth.samhsa.gov/publications/allpubs/ken-01-0104.

Step 6

Check Your Baggage

What Is Baggage?

No one arrives at midlife without baggage. Our past experiences have shaped us, for good and for ill, and can have an impact on our lives in the present. Throughout my interviews the men referred to their baggage—unchanged issues that are not directly related to age or HIV—as well as old concerns, such as seasonal affective disorder, social anxiety, isolation, self-esteem issues, drinking problems, sexual compulsion, and overeating, that affected their ability to adapt to the challenges of aging with HIV.

At their most benign our family histories can lead to patterns of behavior and characteristics that can get us stuck in our ways. Unexamined events in our history can lead to resentments and fears, and can limit flexibility in our current lives. We can develop rigid defenses that impede our growth. Past hurts and traumas can evolve into disorders and compulsions that negatively impact our lives. As you saw in Chapter 9, we become more like ourselves as we grow older. If you do not examine the baggage from your past it can weigh you down.

I cannot know your baggage. That is specific to you. Here I'll present some issues that I have seen in my practice. I will begin with a few of the more serious issues that you must address in order to create your path toward optimal aging with HIV.

Depression

Depression is a general term and can involve either acute episodes of sadness, malaise, and suicidal thought, seasonal depression, or a general feeling of apathy (referred to as dysthymia) that can last for years. Symptoms of depression include diminished interest or pleasure in activities, significant weight loss or gain, insomnia or hypersomnia, psychomotor agitation or retardation, fatigue or loss of energy, feelings of worthlessness or guilt, a diminished ability to think or concentrate, and recurrent thoughts of death. In Chapter 11 you saw how withdrawal, often a symptom of depression, can result in shrinking circles of involvement and stagnation at midlife.

Anxiety

Anxiety can be generalized (affecting you throughout the day) can occur in particular environments (such as social situations and public speaking) or can be acutely felt in the form of panic attacks. Symptoms of anxiety include excessive worry, difficulty in controlling anxious thoughts, feelings of restlessness, being easily fatigued, difficulty concentrating, irritability, muscle tension, sleep disturbance; and impaired social, occupational, or other functioning. When anxiety is untreated it can lead to maladaptive coping strategies and impact your ability to face the challenges of aging with HIV and effectively plan for the future.

Substance Abuse

Throughout the book we identified the negative impact that alcohol and drug abuse can have on your physical health, emotional growth, and optimal aging with HIV. Symptoms of substance abuse include tolerance (a need for more, or a diminished effect of the substance), withdrawal (either physical or psychological), increased use (when the substance is taken in larger amounts or over a longer period than intended), a desire to cut down or unsuccessful efforts to cut down, excessive time spent in activities necessary to obtain or recover from its effects, interference with social, occupational, or recreational activities, and continued use despite knowledge of problems caused by the substance.

Other Disorders

The Diagnostic and Statistical Manual of Mental Disorders[1] lists over 200 conditions that are associated with distress and impairment or disability. Other disorders include posttraumatic stress disorder, obsessive-compulsive disorder, bipolar mood disorders, phobias, and schizophrenia, to name a few. If any of the above concerns are present, I strongly recommend treatment by a licensed mental health professional to address these issues. In the case of addictions, I recommend involvement in a recovery program, including 12-step, inpatient, or outpatient treatment. A detox program may be a good first step, but it is only a short-term solution to a long-term issue.

Low Self-Esteem

Several of the men described how low self-esteem impacted their adaptation to aging with HIV. Low self-esteem can hinder your ability to socialize, reduce your self-confidence in seeking employment, interfere with dating and establishing healthy relationships, sabotage your sex life, and disrupt your self-care strategies. Low self-esteem reduces your self-regard and sense of worth and affects your confidence and sense of efficacy. The challenges of living with HIV and aging can further reduce your self-esteem. Esteem-building exercises, such as affirmations, forming supportive relationships, and recognizing the worth of your accomplishments, can combat low self-esteem.

Other Baggage

Sometimes it can be difficult to identify what is getting in our way. Consider what baggage you have been carrying from your past. Do any of the above issues pertain to you? What other concerns might you face that impede your adaptation to aging with HIV? Is shyness keeping you from meeting new people, pursuing work, or developing relationships? Is cigarette smoking or overeating affecting your physical health? Could compulsive sex be negatively affecting your emotional, spiritual, or financial life? Is the clutter in your home preventing you from inviting people over?

If you need help identifying what obstacles can be interfering with optimal aging you can begin a nightly journal. Write down all the things you did in the day. Include the activities that you wished you could have done differently or that you regret. If you see the same issues arising frequently then you have probably identified the baggage on which you need to work.

Use of Defenses

We all have emotional defenses, and just like physical defenses, we use them to protect ourselves from real or perceived emotional harm. We tend to favor some defenses over others, and mature individuals use defenses flexibly and can select their defenses wisely rather than trigger them compulsively. There is a long list of common defenses, including repression, reaction formation, projection, isolation, undoing, regression, introjection, turning against the self, reversal, sublimation, intellectualization, rationalization, displacement, denial, somatization, idealization, and more. For our purposes it isn't necessary to define all the defenses, but rather to understand that defenses can range from pathological, such as distorting or denying reality when it feels too threatening; to immature, including acting out behaviors without awareness of the motivation; to projection, such as attributing your negative feelings to others; to neurotic, such as avoiding emotions through intellectualization or repression; and, finally, to mature defenses including sublimating your negative emotions into positive actions and identification or modeling yourself after another person's behavior.

The Longitudinal Study of Aging found that the presence of immature defenses at middle age was a contributing factor in poor emotional and physical health in later life.[2] When you use mature defenses you are better equipped to find solutions to your problems, are more adaptive, and are more likely to avoid stagnation at midlife.

Psychotherapy can develop, enhance, modify, and support ego defenses, boosting your ability to use mature defenses. I find that most people come to psychotherapy when their defenses stop working. Usually, they want to be able to make some change in their lives and get back to normal. Sometimes they can make a small change to regain their equilibrium. At other times, the work is deeper and involves internal restructuring—breaking down old defenses and ways of relating to the world while building up new supports, both inside and out.

How Do You Check Your Baggage?

You are never too old to check your baggage and discover a new approach to life. Consider George's story. George had always "enjoyed eating." And he admits he always turned to food as a way to cope with feelings. His weight kept going up and by the time he entered midlife he was overweight. Then the AIDS epidemic began taking all of his friends, and George's overeating became a growing problem. George became obese and despite the warnings he received from doctors, he could not stop eating.

George learned to use food as a way to obtain solace as a child. Both of George's parents were overweight. Now, at 60 years old, George had to face the fact that his weight was having serious effects on his health. He developed a heart condition, he couldn't climb the stairs to his apartment, he was become less active, and dating was "right out of the picture." The future looked bleak.

Then George decided to face this issue from his past and to deal with the impact it was having on his life. George joined Overeaters Anonymous and got back into therapy. He has developed tools to handle his eating and the feelings that trigger the desire to overeat. Today, George is healthier. He can do more physically. His self-esteem is improved. And he is more comfortable being out in the world. He is even considering the possibility of dating.

George's story is not unique. Issues from your past, exacerbated by age and the challenges of life, can serve as impediments to optimal aging with HIV. In order to remove those obstacles you must first identify your baggage and seek out the appropriate path to overcome it.

Some issues are best addressed with a professional psychotherapist. The rationale for reviewing the past in psychotherapy is to uncover the roots of your problems to help you find solutions in the present. A good strategy to find a psychotherapist is to ask for a recommendation from a friend, doctor, or health care provider. You can also contact a local gay or HIV organization for a referral or find one on the web. Some referrals are listed below.

Other issues can be dealt with using a group. In Step 2 we reviewed some guidelines about finding a support group. Support groups provide opportunities for mutual aid, understanding, a universalizing experience, and personal growth. In many self-help groups you are advised to go to six meetings before you determine whether a group is right for you. Go to the resources section of Step 2 to find suggestions for organizations to contact for finding a group.

You may benefit from reviewing self-help books to guide you through a process of healing. A few books to consult are listed under resources.

Obstacles to Checking Your Baggage

You may have many rationalizations as to why you don't need to examine your baggage right now. It is important to determine whether fear is preventing you from getting the most out of your life.

"Psychotherapy is for crazy people." It takes a lot of strength to know you have a problem and courage to seek help. Psychotherapy is for people who are sane enough to know that everyone has issues that they can improve.

"I don't want to pay someone to listen to me." It is great when you have friends who can listen to you. Psychotherapy is not friendship. It is a contract to work on yourself with a trained professional.

"I don't care about other people's problems." Sometimes people wonder whether they will get anything out of joining a group.

The power of mutual aid is sometimes greater than that of individual treatment. Getting to see how you are experienced by others, witnessing other people work through their issues, and having the help of others in solving your problems are powerful forces for individual change and growth.

"*I don't want to dwell in the past.*" Psychotherapy is not about living in the past, but learning from the past to help you in your current life.

"*This is just the way I am.*" It is good to accept yourself. However, you would not say "I have cancer. That's just the way I am." Why do you have to accept changeable aspects of your psychological and emotional health?

It is said that in old age, we become more like ourselves. Midlife is our opportunity to assess our qualities and decide what to take with us into the journey ahead. Continued psychological and emotional growth is an integral part of healthy aging.

Open up your baggage and see what's there. What unaddressed issues from your past are getting in your way? Have you tried to address the problem before? Why didn't it work in the past? Were you ready? Did you choose the wrong approach?

Now may be the time to revisit the issue. Talk to someone else. Ask for help. Try a different approach. Consider professional support. This problem didn't arise overnight, and the solution may not come right away, either.

Resources

Several professional organizations offer websites with referrals for mental health services, including the National Association for Social Workers, www.NASW.org; The Center for Clinical Social Work, www.centercsw.org; and the American Psychological Association, www.apa.org. You can also contact your local chapter of the Center for Clinical Social Work (national website online at www.centercsw.org).

The following books can guide your individual healing:

Don't Call It Love: Recovery from Sexual Addiction by Patrick Carnes

Gay Men at Midlife: Age before Beauty by Alan L. Ellis

Drinking: A Love Story by Caroline Knapp

The Drama of the Gifted Child: The Search for the True Self by Alice Miller

The Road Less Traveled: A New Psychology of Love, Traditional Values and Spiritual Growth by Scott M. Peck

Life After Trauma: A Workbook for Healing by Dena Rosenbloom and Mary Beth Williams

Step 7

Develop Effective Coping Strategies

What Are Effective Coping Strategies?

We all use our own strategies to cope with stress. Whenever we try to solve a problem, call a friend for support, take a deep breath, or have a cry, we are using a coping strategy. Effective coping strategies solve a problem without causing additional stress on your emotional or physical life or negatively affecting your relationships with others. Although some coping strategies are more obviously maladaptive, such as drinking in excess, what makes a strategy effective is its appropriateness for handling a particular situation. Throughout Section I we referred to coping strategies and the need to tailor your approach to your changing needs. For example, in Chapter 1 you identified the coping strategies you used to manage the trauma of learning your HIV status, and you saw how different tools were necessary for dealing with HIV as a chronic illness. And in Chapter 2 you identified the regimens you've developed for living with the physical complications of HIV, reconsidering which were helpful in adapting to age-related changes.

You saw in Chapter 9 how, over the years, you have gotten to know yourself better and have grown to appreciate which coping strategies work best for you. At midlife these tools have become second nature to you and you apply them with little thought. For your coping skills to be most effective, however, you must learn to use them skillfully. Some strategies are better than others in dealing with the problem at hand. You should have a wide variety of tools at your disposal and you need to be flexible in your approach. The use of effective coping strategies is an integral step toward optimal aging with HIV.

Why Are Effective Coping Strategies Important?

In Section II you saw how easy it is to stagnate rather than adapt to aging with HIV. Effective coping is central to avoiding stagnation. You saw how living in the past and relying on old strategies for dealing with the challenges of life do not allow for your changing needs and resources. You also saw how you can get stuck at midlife living within the limitations of aging with HIV. If you are not proactive in seeking out new ways to expand your life you can allow your world to shrink. In Chapter 11 we presented the science concerning locus of control. We demonstrated that people who believe they have greater influence over their lives have better health and well-being at midlife. Developing effective coping strategies enhances your sense of power concerning the things you *can* change.

In Dr. George Vaillant's longitudinal study of aging, the use of effective coping strategies was identified as one of the measures taken at age 50 that best predicted healthy aging at age 70.[1] And effective coping was associated with well-being in a sample of middle-aged and older people living with HIV.[2] As part of a clinical research team at Yale University School of Medicine I tested the effectiveness of a short-term treatment group for middle-aged and older people living with HIV. We added a coping enhancement strategy developed by Folkman and Lazurus[3] to a support group structure. We found that people who completed the coping enhancement protocol evidenced reduced depression and higher levels of physical and emotional well-being.

How Can You Develop Effective Coping Strategies?

There are many strategies for enhancing coping. In the previous step you identified the baggage that could be interfering with your optimal aging with HIV. You considered how psychotherapy, groups, and literature could help you address these issues. Those tools can also be used to enhance your copings strategies. In Chapter 11 you considered your sense of control and applied the serenity prayer to finding solutions. Here is the three-part coping enhancement model we used as part of the Yale study on aging with HIV.

First, you identify your stressor and consider whether it is changeable or unchangeable. A changeable problem (you find out your Medicaid has been cut off, for example) is one that you can do something to address. An unchangeable problem (you've been diagnosed with diabetes) is one you can do nothing to alter.

Second, you develop a plan for dealing with the stressor. If it is changeable, then you choose a problem-focused solution. What can you do to address the stressor? If you've tried everything, talk it over with someone else. A new approach is often the best way to solve a problem-based stressor. If your Medicaid has been cut off there are steps you can take. You can contact the agency that administers Medicaid in your state, get a social worker to help, contact your doctor, or ask a friend for help. These are all problem-focused solutions.

If it is unchangeable, you develop an emotion-focused solution. Examples of unchangeable stressors are losing a friend, dealing with a new diagnosis, or experiencing discrimination. Emotion-focused coping refers to coping strategies aimed at managing or regulating your emotional reaction to a stressor. When we apply emotion-focused coping strategies we engage in an activity that will express, modify, or distract our feelings.

There are many different strategies for emotion-focused coping. It is helpful to know what strategies work best for you, but you should always be developing new coping strategies to help you handle a range of stressors. Also, be aware when coping strategies create new problems. Drinking alcohol, for example, can relax you and help you forget your stress, but drinking in excess can cause other challenges. Even healthy activities, such as exercise, can cause injuries if you are not careful. Here is a short list of emotion-focused coping strategies:

- Meditation, focusing on a single point or image, concentrating on your breathing, or silently repeating a soothing phrase or mantra.

- Using breathing techniques, breathing deeply, or sighing as a way to calm your emotions.
- Visualization, creating an image in your mind of the problem, and solving it. I know someone who visualized a computer game in which the HIV virus was being eaten by gobbling figures. You can also visualize a relaxing place, such as a beach or mountaintop, to soothe yourself.
- Exercise and physical activity can distract you from your stressor, alter your breathing, and revitalize you. In addition, you can visualize your stressor when working out as a way of combating it.
- Taking a walk can help you change your perspective.
- Crying, yelling, and laughing are all good ways to vent your feelings.
- When you reach out to others, either to seek help for your problems or to offer assistance to someone else, you are utilizing emotion-focused coping.
- Journal writing, doing art, dancing, or listening to music are all ways you can creatively express your feelings and reduce your stress.
- Physical activity through aerobics can change your mood; weight training and sports are good outlets for anger.
- Crying, journal writing, and listening to music are all good stress reduction techniques.

There are numerous emotion-focused coping strategies. I am sure that you can think of several that I have left off the list.

Third, you evaluate the effectiveness of the strategy you applied. If it didn't work you try something else. If that, too, is ineffective, maybe you're using the wrong approach. Reconsider whether a problem-based or emotion-based solution would work better. For example, if you are diagnosed with diabetes, you have to cope with this information, and dealing with the feelings that arise from this information. After you've found emotion-focused solutions then there are problem-focused steps to take such as changing your diet, exercising, and taking medications. If you believe you've adapted emotionally to your diagnosis of diabetes, but are finding the regimen of diet and exercise impossible to keep up, reconsider whether you are really coping with your feelings about the diagnosis, or whether feelings of denial, anger, or loss over the diagnosis are causing you to sabotage your efforts to cope.

Most of us do this immediately with little conscious thought. Conscious awareness of your problem-solving approach enhances your coping strategies:

- *Use coping strategies flexibly.* Do not get caught in a pattern of using one or two tools to handle all your problems.
- *Increase the tools at your disposal.* If you need to learn new ways to deal, ask a friend how they would cope in the situation. You can always "borrow" a strategy until it is your own.
- *Be honest.* Sometimes we use strategies that we don't care to admit to, such as eating a box of donuts when we're depressed. And sometimes these strategies work. But when you rely on a strategy that negatively impacts other areas of your life, that's *maladaptive* coping.
- *Reassess regularly.* Periodically review your coping strategies to make sure they are still working.
- *Don't give up.* If the strategy didn't solve the problem, consider why. And then try another approach.

Obstacles to Developing Healthy Coping Strategies

The most frequent obstacle I've encountered while helping people develop effective coping strategies is that they overuse problem-solving methods when emotion-focused coping would be more effective. Trying to get your lover, boss, or landlord to change may seem more satisfying than accepting them as they are, but the only person you have the power to change is yourself. Here are some other obstacles I have encountered in my work.

"I can solve this problem on my own." Knowing when to ask for help is integral to effective coping.

"I'll just deal." When you "get by" you endure difficulties rather than choosing how best to deal with a stressor. Often this means relying on emotional coping strategies when problem-focused strategies might work better.

"I've tried everything and there is nothing I can do." When there is nothing you can do to solve a problem, there is always something you can do to support yourself emotionally.

HIV has taken a great deal away—friends, health, and opportunities. Developing effective coping strategies is empowering and reminds you that you have some control over your life.

Resources

The following books offer some of the best physical and mental techniques that can be used in coping with stress.

The Relaxation and Stress Reduction Workbook by Martha Davis, Matthew McKay, and Elizabeth Eshelman

Mind over Mood: Change How You Feel by Changing the Way You Think by Dennis Greenberger and Christine Padesky

Stress, Appraisal, and Coping by Richard Lazarus and Susan Folkman

The Art of Breathing: Exercises for Improving Your Performance and Well-Being by Nancy Zi

Step 8
Renew Your Spirituality

Why Develop Your Spirituality?

Doctors, mental health practitioners, and social scientists are beginning to recognize what spiritual people have known for years—spirituality can help us with the challenges of illness, aging, addiction, and loss.[1] In Chapter 9 you reviewed the science behind spirituality and how it helps us to mitigate hardships associated with HIV and aging. You identified how your spirituality has evolved over the years. You saw that the spiritual beliefs of your childhood have matured. And you considered when you relied on spiritual practices such as prayer or meditation to help you through crises.

What Does Spirituality Mean to You Today?

Many gay men who have felt ostracized by religious organizations find that the subject of spirituality is filled with complex emotions. Despite philosophical differences, we may still remember the role religion played in our pasts, and we may have a longing for the sense of community, strength, and balance that can come from faith in a higher power. How can we reconcile our inner beliefs with our experiences of alienation, rejection, and oppression?

The men I interviewed have developed creative solutions to this challenge. Some continue to participate in the churches in which they were raised. Some have sought out religions or spiritual practices that they believe accurately represent their personal beliefs. Others have developed individual paths outside the confines of an organized group.

Despite the different approaches, each of the men believes that his spirituality provides a significant form of support. Spiritual beliefs can offer guidance in solving a problem, companionship when we feel alone, solace in times of grief, perspective when we feel overwhelmed, and hope when we are distraught.

Consider what spirituality means to you. Do you have a spiritual practice? Do you participate in an organized religious practice? Do you practice alone or with others? Do you have rituals that you perform on a regular basis or on special occasions? Do you pray or meditate? Do you believe that there is a power greater than yourself? When do you experience that sense or rely on that strength? How did you develop those beliefs?

For many people there is no distinction between spirituality and religion, and for others the two are worlds apart. Your spiritual practice may be informed by religion but also may be completely unique to you.

How Can You Renew Your Spirituality?

I am not an expert on spirituality. I have learned from my interviews that there are innumerable paths to spiritual growth. But there are some common elements to beginning a spiritual practice. I will highlight the tasks that lead us on a spiritual path, using the wisdom of others as a guide.

- *Prayer.* "Ask and you shall receive" is a statement attributed to Jesus Christ. It is an instruction on how to connect ourselves to God. The big book of Alcoholics Anonymous recommends that you pray only for God's will for you and the power to carry that out. The third step prayer can be used to help you connect to a power greater than yourself (replacing the word "God" with Higher Power, good orderly direction, or a symbol that has meaning to you): "God, I offer

myself to Thee—to build with me and to do with me as
Thou wilt. Relieve me of the bondage of self, that I may
better do Thy will. Take away my difficulties, that victory
over them may bear witness to those I would help of Thy
Power, Thy Love, and Thy Way of life. May I do Thy will
always!"[2]

- *Creativity.* Julia Cameron's book *The Artist's Way* is subtitled
  A Spiritual Path to Higher Creativity.[3] In the book she builds
  on spiritual tenets to lead writers, artists, and other people
  who wish to unleash their creativity. And through the
  process of creation, she points out, we draw from a source
  deeper than our individual selves and connect to spiritual
  inspiration.

- *Love.* Transpersonal psychologist and hospice worker
  Dr. Kathleen Dowling Singh explored the spiritual
  development people undergo as they prepare for death. She
  recommends that people at the end of their lives conduct a
  spiritual assessment.[4] What we have learned about love and
  how well we have learned to love are questions included in
  that inventory. Through love of others we can connect to
  our spirituality.

- *Work.* Work can be a path toward spiritual growth,
  connecting you to the universe as a whole. In *The Prophet*
  Kahlil Gibran writes, "When you work you fulfill a part of
  earth's furthest dream, assigned to you when that dream was
  born, and in keeping yourself with labour you are in truth
  loving life."[5]

- *Service.* In *Healthy Aging: A Lifelong Guide to Your Well-Being*,
  Dr. Andrew Weil states that acknowledging and appreciating
  the experience of aging can be a "stimulus for spiritual
  awakening and growth."[6] In his book he offers guidance for
  people seeking to begin a path of spiritual development.
  Among the steps, he states that giving of ourselves can be a
  tool for spiritual growth.

- *Nature.* When we connect with nature we become aware of
  the scale of the universe and realize the size of our lives in
  the process. By experiencing the cycles of life we get to
  know a power beyond ourselves. As Dr. Valliant points out

in his book, *Aging Well*, gardening is a good way to slow down and transcend our individual lives.[7]

• *Faith*. The psychoanalyst Carl Jung referred to synchronicity as evidence of the divine.[8] When serendipitous actions or unusual coincidences occur we are given insight into the workings of the universe. Some people seek guidance in those incongruous events. When we are open to synchronicity in our lives we build a sense of spiritual awareness.

• *Awareness*. When we become aware of our surroundings, leave fantasy behind, and live in the moment we develop spirituality. Jon Kabat-Zinn refers to "being mode"[9] as a way to stop doing anything, not living in the past or thinking ahead to the future. When we can be in the present we can become fully alive.

• *Meditation*. Sri Swami Satchidananda states that meditation begins with concentration—trying to focus your mind on any one point—an idea, word, or form. In the process of meditation your mind will wander, but the constant effort of bringing the mind back again and again to the point of awareness builds concentration and leads to meditation. Meditation is the process by which we get to know our own true selves.[10]

Obstacles to Renewing Your Spirituality

Many people confuse religion with spirituality. There are many diverse forms of spiritual practice. If you believe that you can gain strength from renewing your spirituality then the guidelines offered above can lead you on your individual path toward spiritual development. Define spirituality for yourself, and determine whether a renewed commitment to your beliefs could help you on your path toward optimal aging with HIV.

Your spiritual journey is a unique path. Only you can assess whether you are satisfied by your spiritual life. Could you add depth and meaning to your life by developing or enhancing your daily spiritual practices? Consider your spirituality as part of your overall health.

Resources

The following books provide a variety of modern approaches to spiritual renewal in the individual.

Alcoholics Anonymous: The Story of How Many Thousands of Men and Women Have Recovered from Alcoholism, Third Edition, edited by Alcoholics Anonymous

The Artist's Way: A Spiritual Path to Higher Creativity by Julia Cameron

The Prophet by Kahlil Gibran

Wherever You Go, There You Are: Mindfulness Meditation in Everyday Life by Jon Kabat-Zinn

The Grace In Dying: How We Are Transformed Spiritually as We Die by Kathleen Sing

Meditation by Sri Swami Satchidananda

Aging Well by George Vaillant

Healthy Aging: A Lifelong Guide to Your Well-Being by Andrew Weil

Step 9
Plan for the Future

Why Is It Important to Plan for the Future?

You may have given up planning for the future years ago when AIDS was cutting short the lives of so many of your friends, or when you learned that you were HIV positive. But the transformation of HIV/AIDS from a terminal illness into a chronic condition has enabled you to live longer than you ever expected.

Adapting to aging with HIV means contemplating a future given up to the virus. Throughout Section I you saw the importance of planning. In Chapter 2 you identified the adaptations you need to make to compensate for physical changes as you age. In Chapter 3 you completed an exercise building a corporation of social support for your future self-care needs. In Chapter 8 you identified the financial, emotional, and social needs supplied by work and anticipated how to keep involved in older age. In Chapter 9 you saw how continued growth in later adulthood involves anticipating your future psychological, emotional, and spiritual needs. And in Chapter 13 you recognized that avoiding stagnation and optimizing your aging with HIV involve planning for a future in middle age and beyond.

How Do You Plan for the Future?

To plan for the future, you must first promote a forward-thinking attitude. Planning can be extremely difficult for gay men who have been living with HIV. It is difficult for anyone to plan for an unknown future, but people living with HIV must also be able to put aside fears of mortality sufficiently to conceive of a long life with HIV. You do not know how your HIV status will progress, how your current medication regimen will affect you as you age, and what new treatments will develop. Planning for the future does not mean denying the realities of HIV; rather it means having enough hope to embrace the prospect of living into old age.

To facilitate this new mindset begin with fantasy.

Let's start with a warm-up, "Imaginary Lives," adapted from *The Artist's Way*.[1] This one requires a pen and paper. If you had five other lives to lead what would you do in each of them? I would be a dancer, a stockbroker, a gymnast, a computer engineer, and a performance artist. What would you be if you could have chosen a different path? A football player? A painter? A country singer? A minister? Jot down whatever occurs to you. Do not overthink this exercise. Just have fun imagining different lives for yourself.

Next, dream about your ideal life. Where do you wish you could be in five years? Maybe it is living out one of your imaginary lives. Spend some time letting yourself picture what this new life could be like. Where do you want to live? Who would you spend your time with? What would you want to do in your dream life?

Make up an average day in your dream life from when you wake up in the morning to when (and with whom) you go to bed at night.

Now, let's incorporate some of the things we know about HIV and aging into your fantasies. In five years, who do you want to surround yourself with? Remember, as we get older we have to replace lost friends. That means staying involved socially. Consider where you want to live to maintain and build your social networks. Who is in your social network (friends and family)? How often do you see them? Are there children and young adults in your life? Who do you rely on in case of emergency? How do you get around? Does this ideal life involve a move?

How do you spend your time? As we saw in previous steps, work provides more than just money. It is also a social activity that builds self-esteem and offers opportunities for personal development. Consider what paid or unpaid employment you want to be engaged in. Does your ideal employment match your levels of physical ability? Do you need to learn a new skill or go back to school to succeed? What other activities (hobbies, exercise, making meals, spiritual activities, etc.) are you involved in on a daily basis?

Finally, let's get down to some practical issues to make those dreams come true.

Financial Planning

To meet your goals you need to have the financial means to make them possible. Of course, you could write an entire book on the subject, and many have. Here are some basic guidelines to consider.

First, manage your debt. If you are paying only the minimum due on your credit cards, it will be nearly impossible for you to become free of debt. You may want to contact a credit counselor for ideas on managing your debt.

Second, make a budget and stick to it. Write down your monthly costs (rent/mortgage, food, utilities, entertainment, travel, insurance, medical costs, clothes, miscellaneous). Factor in occasional costs and annual costs. Then check your calculations. Go over your banking statements. Do you spend what you think you do? Do you live within your means? Can you add money to savings? What would happen if your income were affected by illness or other factors? Are you dependent on someone else's income?

Third, plan for retirement. If you have a pension you are among the very few left with a clear sense of how much money you will have when you retire. For the rest of us, we must do a great deal of calculating and hopeful thinking. The Social Security Administration annually sends out a statement indicating the benefits you would receive if you were to become disabled and indicating what your rate of payment will be upon retirement. Retirees can start receiving benefits from Social Security at age 62. Remember, when you retire "early" the benefit is reduced. To receive your full Social Security retirement benefit you must be age 65 and 10 months if you were born in 1942. Anyone born in years 1943 through 1954 must be 66 years old and those born in 1960 and later must be 67 years of age to receive full benefits.

If you have additional funds, you should be thinking about investing for retirement. There are calculators on the web to determine how much you must contribute to your retirement plan to reach certain monetary goals. Much of retirement planning has to do with risk, and many financial counselors recommend that your risk should decrease as you age. Consider consulting an expert. The resources section has some recommendations on where to go for financial advice.

Fourth, consider whether you need insurance to protect your assets. Aside from health insurance, which we will discuss later, there are many types of insurance, such as homeowners', renters', auto, life, and disability. As Suze Orman explains, insurance is "a bet between you and the insurance company ... usually the company is right."[2] Think about whether having insurance will offer you peace of mind.

Medical Insurance

Here, too, we've entered into a complex and ever changing arena. We are currently in an era of health care reform, and therefore changes may occur affecting the insurance industry, Medicare, and other health-related programs. Currently, many of us rely on health insurance policies to cover our medical expenses. You may have private medical insurance offered through your employer. In that case, your premium may be offset by participating in a group plan. Choosing the right plan is often a challenge as you need to make decisions based on the premium, deductibles, and coverage. What may seem the least expensive plan in the short run may become far more expensive given your monthly medical and prescription expenses or the event of a hospitalization. There are many types of insurance plans, including Health Maintenance Organizations (HMO), Preferred Provider Organizations (PPO), and Point of Service Plans (POS). You can choose to purchase a plan as an individual person—the rates are then much higher. Or you can join a group plan based on a professional organization (for example, the Freelancers Union offers insurance plans at a group rate). When you leave a job you can elect to continue your insurance for a period of 18 months under the COBRA act, which may be less expensive than buying your own individual policy.

Medicare is available to anyone who receives Social Security Disability or is over the age of 65. In most cases there is no charge for Medicare Part A (if you did not contribute through work, however, the premium is quite high) and a monthly premium for Part B. Part A covers hospital care, skilled nursing, home care, and hospice care. Part B covers physician's services, outpatient care, physical therapy, and ambulance care. Neither covers dental care, vision care, or medication costs. Each plan has necessary deductibles that you must meet annually and Part A has a co-payment for hospital stays. You are automatically enrolled in Medicare at age 65, but can opt out of Part B, if you choose.

You can also enroll in a Medicare Health Plan offered by a private insurance carrier (HMO or PPO). The Medicare.gov website explains: "They generally offer extra benefits, and many include pre-scription drug coverage. These plans often have networks, which means you may have to see doctors who belong to the plan or go to certain hospitals to get covered services. In many cases, your costs for services can be lower than in Original Medicare, but it is important to check with the plan because the costs for services will vary."[3]

You can enroll in a Medicare prescription coverage plan (Medicare Part D), an AIDS Drug Assistance Program (ADAP) administered by your state, or both to cover the cost of prescrip-tion drugs. To obtain more information about Part D go to their website at www.medicare.gov/pdp-basic-information.asp. To compare Medicare and ADAP coverage go to the federal govern-ment website at www.hrsa.gov/partdhiv/adap.htm. Or for more information about ADAP, you must contact the department of health in your state or talk to your doctor or social worker.

There are also currently 12 different types of supplemental insurance plans (Medigap Plans) that you can purchase to cover costs that Medicare doesn't. They are offered through private insurance carriers and are labeled with letters A–L. A is the most basic, and increased and varied benefits are included in the other available plans. You are advised to review them all before deciding which is best for you. Remember, no matter which insurance com-pany offers a particular plan, all plans with the same letter cover the same benefits. For instance, all Plan C policies have the same benefits no matter which company sells the plan. However, the premiums can vary.

Medicaid covers medical care for poor Americans. People also apply for Medicaid to cover costs when there is extreme need, especially in terms of long-term care. Medicaid coverage is compli-cated and varies by state. For example, in New York State you can be allocated Medicaid coverage based on a spend down analysis. Depending on your medical expenses, you can be covered for a period of one to several months. You must pay close attention to your Medicaid coverage to avoid having your coverage discontinued.

Finally, you can purchase a long-term care policy to cover the expenses of medical, social, or support services needed over a long period of time. These expenses are often not covered by Medicare, Medicaid, and Medigap policies.

As you can see, medical insurance is a complicated issue. And given your HIV status, you should talk to an expert about what you are eligible for and which policies are most appropriate for you. See the section on resources, below, for more advice.

Legal Issues

There are some legal issues to consider as you age with HIV. Gay marriage, although it has become legal in some states, does not offer the same legal benefits as heterosexual marriage in the United States. Therefore, you will need to make sure that your assets are protected if you are in a committed relationship. Cohabitation agreements, bank account titles, and the writing of titles and deeds are important issues for same-sex couples to consider. I recommend going to a lawyer for expert advice in this area. I have also included a guide on legal planning for same-sex couples in the resources section.

In the case of your illness you will want someone to have a health care proxy. Have you discussed your wishes with a friend or family member? Depending on the state in which you live they may need a legal document, such as a health care proxy, living will, or power of attorney, to make decisions about your medical care and to have access to your finances.

You will need to write a legal will to make sure that your assets are allocated according to your wishes when you die. These papers can be downloaded from the web, but in many states they are not entirely enforceable unless they are written by a lawyer. Estate planning is particularly important for gay couples who are not equally protected under the law. If you are in a relationship, you need to consult a lawyer in your state to make sure that your partner can inherit your estate without conflict or an unnecessary tax burden. The resources section below will help you find the information you need to protect yourself and your partner.

It has been my experience that people postpone completing these important documents, sometimes until it is too late, because they do not want to consider the realities of their illness and death. We are all going to die. Managing these concerns should give you the freedom to live your life, knowing that you have taken care of your responsibilities and seen that your wishes will be carried out.

Translate Your Fantasies into a Real Life Plan

Now, integrate these practical issues into the dream life discussed at the beginning of this chapter and write a five year plan. Make a list of goals that you would like to accomplish within the next five years. They may be large, such as get a college degree, or smaller, like clean out the hall closet. Put them all down on paper.

Select five goals and list them separately. Leave space between each to enumerate the objectives you need to accomplish to reach each goal. What steps do you need to take to complete the task? Now create a reasonable time line to accomplish each task and meet your goal. You will need to be flexible. You might find that the task is more difficult than you anticipated, or there may be changes in your life that reshape your goal. Having deadlines can be a good motivator, but don't be rigid. You can become overwhelmed and give up if you are not open to changes in your health, needs, and environment.

Select one goal to start working on today. Review this list frequently. See if you are meeting your targets, and, if not, figure out what is getting in the way. When you have completed all five goals listed on the paper pull five more from your first list. Over time you will see what you have achieved, what you still have to do, and what you want to add to that list.

Obstacles to Planning for the Future

When planning for the future we can get caught in two ruts.

One, we have rich fantasies, but we do not follow through on our plans. The list, once written, should be referred to often. Stick to your goals.

Two, we get caught up in the practicalities of daily life and do not envision a plan for ourselves. Fantasy can be a font of information. When we let ourselves dream we learn about ourselves and our desires. We can choose to act on the information that our fantasies have to offer.

Some excuses I have heard to avoid planning include the following.

"*I don't know if I'll live that long.*" You've probably lived longer than you expected, so don't be so sure. Planning for the future involves preparing for possibilities. Once you start on the path you may change the journey, but you need to begin somewhere.

"*I'll be fine.*" You probably will be. But to make the most out of your life, you need a vision for yourself. Relying on the universe to take care of you is passive and doesn't give you the opportunities to make the most out of your future. See what is behind your inactivity. You may find that your easygoing attitude may be covering fear.

"*I have too much to do already.*" Getting caught up in the day-to-day can cloud your overall vision for your life. The activities you are working on today may fit into a larger plan. Remember, you do not need a *perfect* plan for aging with HIV, only an *optimal* plan that includes all the realities and challenges to make the most of your future.

"*It's too late.*" It is never too late to start a new life—or to renew your old one. Every day you allow fear, hesitation, and inertia to hold you back you are preventing yourself from finding your optimal path toward aging with HIV.

"*I live life one day at a time.*" Living one day at a time is a wonderful strategy for life at its fullest. However, you can live one day at a time and still plan for the future. When you have a life plan that can accommodate internal and external changes you can allow yourself to live more fully in the present knowing that your life has direction.

Having a flexible life plan is an integral part of optimal aging with HIV. Planning involves accepting and embracing an unknown future living with HIV, recognizing and adapting to your limitations, and responding to your desires. Review your life plan and make sure it has been adapted to the changes of aging with HIV, recognizes your current needs, and anticipates future challenges.

Resources

Knowledge is the key to good planning. There is a lot to consider and if you are not good at numbers, like me, you can become overwhelmed and give up when it comes to financial, legal, and health care planning. Try to digest the information a piece at a time. Here are some places to find expert advice in each area:

Financial: www.gfn.com (the gay financial network) has articles and referrals. I also recommend *The Road to Wealth: A Comprehensive Guide to Your Money* and other books by Suze Orman for financial planning.

Legal: www.lawhelp.org offers referrals and recommendations throughout the United States. Lambda Legal has a comprehensive life planning tool kit on their website at www.lambdalegal.org. One helpful resource is the book *A Legal Guide for Lesbian and Gay Couples*, by Denis Clifford, Frederick Hertz, Robin Leonard, and Hayden Curry.

Health care: AARP has information on health care plans, long-term care insurance and Medicare on their website at www.aarp.org.

Step 10

Play

Why Does Play Matter?

It may seem out of place to end a book on aging with HIV by discussing play. But the ability to play is probably one of the most influential factors in development across the lifespan, and it is an integral step toward optimal aging with HIV.

Most of what we know as adults we learned through play as children. But as we age we often forget the importance of playtime. Think of the ways you grew from play.

When you were little did you ever go up to a stranger and ask, "Do you want to play?" Playtime helps us make new friends and teaches us socialization skills.

Did you make up games, draw, or build things when you played by yourself or with others? Through play we let our fantasy life take shape and channel our creativity into action. Creativity could distract us from loneliness and help us interact with others in new ways. Imaginative play was the inspiration for our future work. Through creative play we shaped our growing minds.

Think about all the competitive games you played as a kid—"duck, duck, goose," board games and cards, make believe, and organized sports. Through competitive play we learn to handle defeats and victories on the playground that would help us manage wins and losses in later life. Some active competition also got our heart rate up with needed physical activity.

Finally, there was endless learning through play. We learned how to handle money through counting games, to spell and read through word games, and even to get to know the human body from playing doctor. The great thing about most of these games is that we were learning while we were having fun.

Considering all that you gained through play as children, how can you benefit from play at this life stage? In Chapter 8 you identified four benefits of work that need to be present in a rewarding retirement. Not coincidentally, they are socializing, expressing creativity, physical or intellectual competition, and life-long learning. Finding avenues for play can keep us physically and intellectually stimulated, socially involved, and offer opportunities for continued emotional development, all of which can counteract stagnation and increase adaptation at midlife and beyond.

How Can You Play at This Age?

Do you play enough? In Chapter 8 you completed an assignment in which you listed five benefits of play and identified how you can recreate these activities in your life today. Review those hobbies, physical activities, and creative and social engagements, and make sure that play is well represented.

Organized sports can be great forms of play, when they are not taken too seriously, and are not beyond your physical capabilities. When you are involved in a strenuous sport you get much-needed exercise and increase your endorphins. In team sports, such as basketball, you stay connected to others. You can play golf alone or with friends. And, bowling is a lower energy sport that can still work up a sweat. Even if you are not an athlete, you can find a sport that isn't too intimidating. Jogging, rowing, bicycling, and kayaking are all independent sports that have meditative qualities. Less conventional sports such as ballet, ballroom dance, fencing, and yoga are all forms of play. Games such as cards, Scrabble™, and board games have the same opportunities for competitive activity, intellectual challenge, and socialization without the strain of physical activity.

Creative activities can be done alone or with others. Making art, writing, woodworking, and gardening are all creative activities in which you participate in making something new. Do you enjoy listening to music? Dancing to rock and roll or drums? Cooking, needlework, collecting? You can take a class to learn a new hobby or skill. Join an improvisation group. Care for animals. Any of these activities can broaden your sense of creative play.

If you need help developing your ability just spend time with a child. My biggest pleasure is watching a child who has just opened a present make a toy out of the box it came it. You can invent play from your imagination, too.

Obstacles to Playing

"I've got no talents." You do not have to be good at an activity to enjoy it.

"It's too late for me to develop hobbies." You can always learn a new skill, and you may find that you are better than you anticipated. Anyway, the fun lies in the process of learning.

"Being an artist—that's just egocentric." Participating in creative activities is an expression of something beyond the individual. Sharing your creativity with others is a gift.

"People will think I'm weird." People may, but they may also admire you. Normalcy is overrated.

"I have too much to do." Play is serious business—an outlet for physical activity, socializing, stress reduction, and emotional and psychological development. Play should be part of your health care regimen.

Laughter is good medicine. Start having some fun! Doctor's orders.

Resources

The Artist's Way: A Spiritual Path to Higher Creativity by Julia Cameron

Conclusion

With treatment for HIV disease, gay men are living longer then they ever expected, but as you know, there is a difference between surviving and thriving. For all of us, aging involves adapting to a myriad of changes. However, the challenges of the AIDS epidemic and its impact on your personal life, your body, your family, your friends, and your communities have knocked you off course in your adaptation to aging with HIV.

Your hard work in completing the exercises in *Aging with HIV: A Gay Man's Guide* has helped you gain insight and take steps to optimize your life. First, you reviewed how aging means changes in your life. Through a review of the research, reading the men's narratives, and completing a series of exercises you reassessed your experience of aging across nine fields of life: the course of the AIDS epidemic, alterations in your body, changing friendship networks, developing a new place in the gay community, developing a new attitude about sex, experiencing changing relationships, experiencing new roles in the family, developing a new approach to work, and internal changes. Only by identifying the changes you have undergone were you then able to assess your adaptation to those changes.

In Section II you examined where you might have gotten stuck along the way. You answered four questions to evaluate your experience of aging. You considered whether you are learning from the past or living in the past, living within limits or letting your world shrink, accepting yourself or getting stuck in your ways, and living one day at a time or relinquishing a plan for the future. Through a thorough self-examination you saw areas of your life that you needed to change to make the most out of this phase of your life.

Finally, you completed the steps toward optimal aging with HIV. In the third section you developed new skills and reworked old tools to move forward, with flexibility and strength, to make the most of your current life and meet the challenges ahead. The 10 steps toward optimal aging with HIV are to care for your physical health; rebuild your social networks; be generative; fight the triple threat of the AIDS stigma, homophobia, and ageism; let yourself grieve; check your baggage; develop effective coping strategies; renew your spirituality; plan for the future; and play.

It was quite an undertaking. I hope you appreciate how far you've come and that you've taken good care of yourself along the way, taking breaks, getting plenty of rest, and asking for support when it was needed. You may have skipped over sections, found that certain questions or exercises didn't work for you, and found your own ways to evaluate your experience. That's okay. Remember, aging with HIV is new territory, and you are discovering your unique path toward optimal aging.

You may want to check back with these exercises periodically. Questions that had little relevance may become more significant over time. You can also return to the book to reflect on your progress, to see if you are still on track, or to assess how you are coping with new challenges that arise.

The research on HIV and aging is ever expanding, and new findings may reshape our current understanding. You will have to keep abreast of what is out there and reconsider whether the suggestions in this book remain relevant over time. Your experience in completing this book should have given you the tools to process new developments, assess their impact on your life, and adapt to changes as you age with HIV.

I hope that this book has helped you to appreciate your aging body, mind, and spirit, and that your increased curiosity and interest have led to finding new ways to care for yourself. Optimal aging with HIV means making the most of this phase of your life, adapting to changes one day at a time, and balancing the need to reflect on the past, live in the present, and plan for the future. I wish you a fulfilling journey on your continuing path to optimal aging with HIV.

About the Study

The Study

The model for optimal aging presented in this book emerged from a study conducted at and funded through New York University School of Social Work, as well as a fellowship from the John A. Hartford Foundation.

Background

The study was developed to respond to three dynamics found in the literature: the large and growing number of people aging with HIV, the evidence that older adults experience higher rates of mortality and morbidity than younger adults living with HIV, and the knowledge gap between research in this area and gerontological theory.

Rates of HIV/AIDS diagnosis in the United States are experiencing the greatest increase among those in the 50- to 64-year-old age group. The percentage of those diagnosed with AIDS over age 50 has increased from 10% in the period from 1993 to 1995 to 12.3% in the period from 1996 to 2000, and it is estimated that presently this proportion may be close to 20%.[1]

Research on middle-aged and older adults living with HIV has found that this group has higher rates of mortality than younger people with the virus.[2] This group has also evidenced elevated levels of depression and anxiety, reduced quality of life, and significant limitations related to poor finances, lack of social support, stigma, and discrimination.[3] In contrast to these findings, middle-aged and older people living with the virus have described age as both an advantage and a disadvantage in living with HIV.[4]

The majority of research on HIV has studied all people 50 and older as one age group. Yet Linsk[5] found that there are several age cohorts among gay men over 50 living with HIV, a conclusion supported by the gerontological literature.[6]

In response to the growing population of gay men aging with HIV, the special concerns raised by the research on this community, and the need to apply gerontological knowledge to the study of aging with HIV, this study was designed to explore, examine, and understand the experience of aging for a group of gay men living with HIV in late middle age.

Methodology

This study was designed to answer the following research questions.

1. How do gay men in late middle age construct the experience of aging with HIV/AIDS?
2. What meanings do they attribute to aging? How do they relate their experience of aging to having HIV/AIDS? How do they relate their experience of aging to their sexuality?
3. What role do themes from the research on gay men's aging at middle age (i.e., physical changes, relationships, work, loss, accelerated aging, crisis competence, stigma, and the importance of the gay community) play in gay men's experience of living with HIV/AIDS? How is the concept of generativity reflected in their experience?

Rationale for the Methodology

The choice of a qualitative approach reflected the intention to learn about the "lived experience"[7] of this underresearched population. Qualitative methods involve an in-depth exploration of a phenomenon, and are chosen when there is interest in how people interpret their experiences, how they construct their worlds, and what meaning they attribute to their experiences.[8] Minimally structured interviews of a small set of individuals allow for a "thick description"[9] of a phenomenon. Qualitative methods are selected when little is known about a population or topic, when pursuing a topic of sensitivity and emotional depth, when one wishes to gain insight into the perspectives of individuals, and when quantitative data are insufficient for developing understanding. Exploratory methods and the qualitative paradigm are also recommended when studying hidden or stigmatized populations. As discussed in earlier sections, the triple threat of ageism, homophobia, and HIV/AIDS stigma has significantly affected this community; the subject matter is sensitive and the goal of this study has been to develop an in-depth understanding of these men's experience. Therefore, the nature of the population, the subject, and the study purpose have dictated the use of the study method.

The qualitative methods used here are nested in a tradition of grounded theory and methods. The distinguishing characteristics of grounded theory include simultaneous involvement in data collection and analysis; creation of analytic codes and categories developed from the data, not from preconceived hypotheses; the development of axial codes, middle-range theories that influence both the development of theory and the analysis of codes; memo making, writing analytic notes to explicate and fill out categories; theoretical sampling; and delay of the literature review.[10] The strength of this method lies in its ability to capture and make sense of the complexity of the phenomena studied.

Participant Sampling, Characteristics, and Recruitment

Study participants met the following inclusion criteria: (1) age 50 to 64 years, (2) a self-reported HIV-positive serostatus or diagnosis of AIDS, (3) male, (4) self-identification as gay, (5) English speaking, and (6) provision of informed consent. Participants were self-selecting and responded to a flier that clearly stated the recruitment criteria. A screening form was used to determine eligibility.

Because the aim was to study the breadth of experience within the defined population, purposive sampling was used to gather a diverse sample according to race, age, and health within the study parameters, with no assumptions about how this diversity might affect responses. Purposive sampling is the selection of participants based on their ability to provide a comprehensive understanding of the subject, who can elicit data on emergent theory.[11] The suspected mode of HIV transmission was not considered in recruitment, and persons with a history of substance use were included. Participants who seroconverted before the onset of middle age as well as those who became positive after becoming middle aged were included. Men throughout the spectrum of HIV/AIDS (from HIV asymptomatic to AIDS diagnosis) were included. Differences according to race, age, and other variables are noted in a demographic chart. The ultimate sample size of 15 was determined by the richness of the data.

Participants were primarily recruited from SAGE (called "Senior Action in a Gay Environment" at the time of the study; now known as Services and Advocacy for Gay, Lesbian, Bisexual, and Transgender Elders) New York, a social service organization in the gay community. Fliers were posted on the SAGE bulletin boards within the Lesbian and Gay Community Services Center to provide access to a large number of individuals. During the data collection phase it became apparent that "word of mouth" or unintentional snowball sampling had expanded recruitment. The 15 respondents lived in four of the five boroughs of New York City (there were no respondents from Staten Island). And interviews were conducted in a range of housing environments, from projects and SROs to expensive cooperative apartment buildings.

Data Collection

The data collection period began in August 2004. This study received approval from the Human Subjects Review Committee at New York University and respondents gave signed consent. Data were coded and names of participants as well as any identifying information were changed. Participants each received $20 cash compensation per interview. The data collection consisted of a telephone screening interview, an initial audio-taped interview in the participant's home lasting approximately 90 minutes, and audio-taped follow-up and member checking interviews of varied lengths.

During the audio-taped interview, participants were encouraged to tell their own story and, using an interview checklist as a guide, I "followed the lead" of respondents, asking questions to elucidate and expand on emergent data.

Data Analysis

A systematic strategy of data analysis consistent with grounded theory was employed, as outlined above. Open coding was used to identify meaning units directly from the data, rather than a priori concepts. First, I used a strategy of line-by-line coding—examining each line of the data and identifying key words, phrases, or statements. Using constant comparative analysis, codes were compared between the data of single interviews and across interviews, merged, deleted, created, and moved. Axial coding was used to relate codes and create code families. Throughout the data analysis process I created memos in the text, noting ideas prompted from the interviews. Memos were aggregated along with codes using a computer software program, ATLAS-TI.[12] Journal entries logged coding decisions and recorded overall impressions or themes.

Enhancing Rigor

I have incorporated Padgett's[13] six strategies for enhancing rigor in qualitative research.

- *Audit Trail.* Journal entries, field notes, as well as face sheets and transcribed interviews comprise the audit trail, and can be used to determine intrarater reliability.
- *Peer Debriefing.* I participated in a qualitative research peer debriefing and support group (PDS).
- *Triangulation of Data.* There are several forms of data that can be used to corroborate or challenge findings, including transcription of interviews, face sheets, extensive field notes,

journal entries, documents, and notes from attendance at a forum on Gay Aging at Middle Age.
* *Prolonged Engagement.* Multiple interviews have been conducted over the course of 18 months.
* *Member Checking.* During member checking interviews I asked participants to comment on specific ideas arising from their interviews.
* *Negative Case Analysis.* I examined the findings to look for evidence that either disproved emergent theory or refined it.

Limitations

Although the research involved strategies to enhance rigor, there are some limitations to this current study. Recruitment was successful in including a diverse pool of participants involved with more than one social service organization, but recruitment efforts reached participants who are probably more integrated into formal social support systems than is representative of this group as a whole. Recruiting from the New York City area may also have omitted individuals who are more geographically isolated. Recruitment procedures, reaching out to individuals who speak English fluently and who are interested in participating in this interview, as well as the nature of qualitative inquiry that relies on individuals who can tell their story in a cogent manner may have attracted individuals who may not represent the demographics of this population as a whole and who may be healthier, wealthier, and more educated. Sampling could have produced an unknown level of homogeneity with a subset of participants (e.g., friendship networks). Finally, there have been potential effects, endemic to the field of qualitative study, in the use of myself as the research instrument and my impact on the interaction with participants.

This study was intended to be an initial exploration and development of theory on aging with HIV/AIDS among gay men at middle age. The theory developed from this study has focused on the role of adjustment to aging with HIV/AIDS in the lives of gay men at middle age. The findings on adjustment are exploratory and it is my hope that future research will be able to expand on these findings and consider, and possibly ameliorate, some of its limitations.

Results

A total of 71 codes emerged from the data; 22 axial codes were identified and 3 selective codes or themes were developed. A few open codes were represented in more than one code family.

The three themes formed the basis of the emergent theory, Adaptation vs. Stagnation. They were Traversing Fields of Change, Orientation to Time, and Contributing Factors. Chart A presents a concept map for Theme I and demonstrates the evolution from codes to axial codes and themes.

Theme I: Adapting to change was a central theme throughout the interviews. Frequently used phrases such as "a new phase," "turning point," and "double change" underscored the significance of the theme of change in their lives, whereas concepts such as "new approach," "reassess," and "changing priorities" emphasized the importance of adaptation. The men identified eight areas in which aging with HIV involved adaptation to change. They were redefining being gay, the course of the HIV/AIDS epidemic, changing friendship networks, new roles in the family, changing sex lives and intimate relationships, a new relationship to work and career, and physical and internal changes.

Theme II: Orientation to time also played an important role in the interviews. The men presented time-related challenges, including the decision to "live in the past," "learn from the past," or "put things in the past." A similar dialectic emerged between "living one day at a time" and "planning for the future." Several of the men noted that over time their lives had gotten smaller, what Mario refers to as "a shrinking kind of life."

Theme III: The third theme identified the factors that can both assist with or impede adaptive aging with HIV. Frequently used phrases such as "your approach to surviving," "the key to my survival," and "that's what helped me cope" demonstrated that the men had identified strategies to adapt to aging with HIV. Nine contributing factors were identified: historical factors, internal

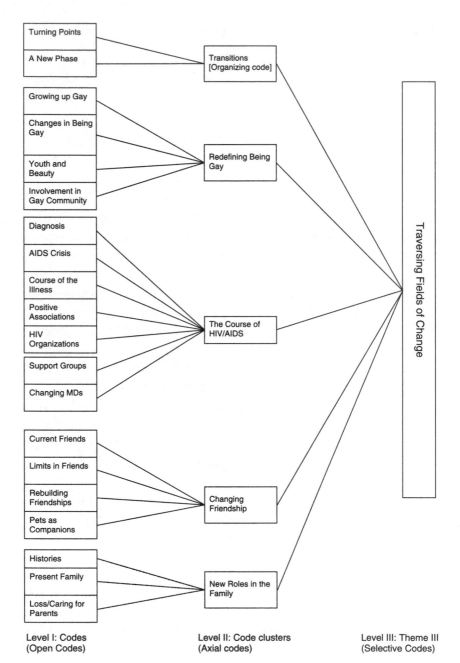

Level I: Codes	Level II: Code clusters	Level III: Theme III
(Open Codes)	(Axial codes)	(Selective Codes)

Chart A. Codes and Code Clusters for Theme I (Traversing Fields of Change).

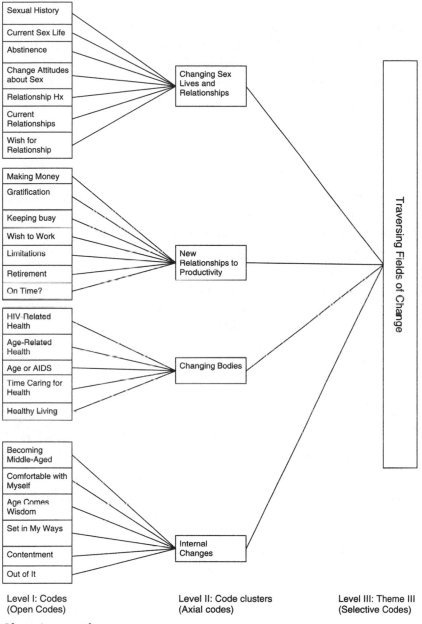

| Level I: Codes | Level II: Code clusters | Level III: Theme III |
| (Open Codes) | (Axial codes) | (Selective Codes) |

Chart A. cont'd

resources, resilience, external resources, physical health, AIDS stigma, feelings about aging, mortality, and sense of agency.

The book *Aging with HIV: A Gay Man's Guide* presents the findings of the study in an accessible format. The codes, axial codes, and themes are presented as quotes, chapters, and sections of the book.

Conclusion

The overarching theme, adaptation versus stagnation, emerged from the analysis of the data. The study found that adaptation to change was the most salient feature of aging with HIV for gay men at middle age. Gay men in midlife have lived longer than they expected and must adapt to changes within their interpersonal and internal worlds. Although many of these changes (physical changes or work or family) are common for other men in their age group,[14] HIV-positive men who thought they would not live to middle age have not anticipated the challenges of aging and have not had the mirroring and support of a cohort of their peers, many of whom died in the AIDS epidemic, to help them anticipate, manage, and adapt to the "normal" transitions of aging.

The threat of stagnation in this period is real, and can be evidenced in behaviors such as living in the past and letting their worlds shrink. For the most part, gay men living with HIV at midlife are aware of these challenges and can identify the factors that contribute to their adaptation to aging. However, adaptation is an elusive concept. And the study finds that adapting to aging with HIV is a multidimensional dynamic, involving the ability to appraise one's life, reassess strategies and supports, and develop new tools that adjust to changing situations across several spheres of life.

The significant role that emotions can play in either impeding or enhancing adaptation to aging with HIV was, perhaps, the most salient result of this study. I found that unacknowledged and unaddressed emotions, such as grief, stigma, survivor guilt, and shame, act as barriers to optimal aging with HIV, preventing the adoption of self-care strategies and aiding in the creation of a shrinking kind of life.

In order to avoid stagnation and make the most of aging with HIV at midlife, gay men must adapt to the myriad of life changes associated with aging with HIV. This involves confronting internal and external obstacles, maintaining and building social supports, integrating the past, living in the present, and reclaiming a future previously relinquished to AIDS.

The strategies presented in *Aging with HIV: A Gay Man's Guide* evolved from my discussions with these men, the HIV and aging literature, and over 20 years of experience in the field. It is my hope that this book can be a tool to help gay men living with HIV, and the people who care for them, in their path toward optimal aging.

Using This Book in a Group

Here is a brief outline on how to use the material in this book in a support group format.

Pregroup Planning

Purpose: Taking some time to prepare for your new group can give you the opportunity to anticipate challenges and take steps to enhance the group's success. Some of the following issues should be considered:

- Membership—Who will be invited to join the group and how will they be recruited (word of mouth, flier, an existing group)? How many members? (I often begin a group when I have at least 6 people to start, but I aim for 8 to 10 members.) How much diversity (race, age, background, etc.) of membership will assist in the discussion and encourage growth?
- Leadership—Will there be a professional facilitator? Peer leaders? Will the leadership remain constant or rotate? Will there be more than one facilitator? If you are forming a peer-led group I recommend having a psychotherapist available for consultation or referral if the need arises.
- Location—Where will the group meet? If at an agency or organization is the space confirmed for the full run of the group? If at someone's home, what will happen if they

drop out? Is the space conveniently located, well lit, quiet, and comfortable?

- Structure/content—There are many ways to run a group. I recommend beginning each session with a check-in go around, moving into the exercise, and leaving time for feedback at the end. You should begin to think about what structure will work best for your group.
- Group rules—Following with guidelines will ensure that the time is shared and that all people feel safe and comfortable. Among the issues to consider are confidentiality, tardiness, attendance, respect, how to handle conflict, and whether cross-talk is allowed. These issues will be ironed out with the group members during the group's first meetings.

Week 1: Introductions

Purpose: Getting to know each other and the group as a whole.

The group leader(s) will begin by stating why they formed the group and will then go around the room asking each member why they are there and what they hope to gain from the experience.

After a brief statement about confidentiality the group members will start laying down the group rules (see pregroup planning). I advise limiting the time of this discussion. Unresolved issues can be revisited next week.

Members are encouraged to tell their stories. The following questions can be used to prompt discussion: What does aging with HIV mean to you? How do you feel about growing older? See the preface for additional questions. Or you can follow up on points made in the initial go around.

Wrap-up. What did you get out of the first meeting? What did you hope to get that you didn't get? Will you come back? What issues are still on the table for next week?

Homework: Read Chapter 1 and complete the assignment.

Weeks 2–10: Aging Means Changing

Purpose: Using the book as a guide, you will join each other in a reevaluation of your lives, identifying the changes, sometimes shared, sometimes unique to each member, that you have under-gone as you have been aging with HIV.

Check-in: How did you feel about last week's session? How are you feeling about being here today? Are there any unresolved issues to discuss?

Discuss any issues from the previous week.

Discuss the chapter and assignment. Group members may want to bring in their homework, work on it in the group, or discuss their overall impressions from the reading.

Wrap up and review the session, see how people are doing, and choose the homework assignment for the following week.

Week 10 homework assignment: Read all of Section II, answer-ing questions and completing assignments on your own. Once you have identified how you have gotten stuck in your adaptation to aging with HIV, be prepared to talk about it in the group.

Weeks 11 and 12: Identify Challenges

Purpose: Group members will help each other identify the common and unique ways each has gotten stuck in their adaptation to aging.

Follow the same format as weeks 1–10 (check-in go around, unresolved issues, discussion, and wrap-up).

The discussion of "getting stuck" will be more free-flowing, as members should be more comfortable with the group process. Leaders can refer to questions and exercises from the chapters to facilitate the discussion. Each member will be encouraged to iden-tify at least one area of his life in which he feels that he has been stagnating.

Homework: Read Section III.

Weeks 13 and 14: Steps toward Optimal Aging

Purpose: The group members will develop strategies to help each other find his own path toward optimal aging with HIV and to use the group sessions to set clear goals and objectives.

Use the discussion time to develop a five year plan with the help of the group. Come up with a vision for your future and determine what steps you need to take to make those goals a reality. Use the exercise in Step 9 as a guide. Participants can help each other by giving feedback and providing ideas and encouragement.

If you have more time, you can extend the group's process. In a six-month group, weeks 13–14 can be expanded to ten weeks. Each meeting can address one step, helping each other utilize the steps in your daily lives.

Weeks 15 and 16: Goodbyes

Purpose: The group has been through a unique process together and members should take the time to review what they have accomplished, reflect on the help they have received, and anticipate the support and tools they need to continue the work on their own.

Some of the following questions should be considered during the termination phase: Did you get what you expected? How have you grown? What will you take with you from this experience? What will you do with this time now that the group is ending? Identify one person who touched you in the group. Tell him how he made a difference in your life. Even if you decide to stay in touch informally, this is the end of your relationships in the group. Make sure you say goodbye to each member and to the group as a whole.

Notes

PREFACE

1. All names and identifying information have been changed to maintain confidentiality.

2. NCHS Data Warehouse on Trends in Health and Aging. (2004). Trends in HIV/AIDS in Aging Americans. www.cdc.gov/nchs/agingact.htm.

3. Centers for Disease Control (2010) Diagnoses of HIV Infection and AIDS in the United States and Dependent Areas, 2008; *HIV Surveillance Report*, Volume 20, June 14, 2010; http://www.cdc.gov/hiv/surveillance/resources/reports/2008report/index.htm.

4. Gabriel, M. A. (1996). *AIDS Trauma and Support Group Therapy: Mutual Aid, Empowerment, Connection*. New York: The Free Press.

5. Heckman, T., Kochman, A., Sikkema, K. J., Kalichman, S. C., Masten, J., Bergholte, J., & Catz, S. (2001). A pilot coping improvement intervention for late middle aged and older adults living with HIV/AIDS in the USA. *AIDS, 13*(1), 129–139.

6. Masten, J. E. (2007). *Aging with HIV/AIDS: The Experience of Gay Men in Late Middle Age*. Ann Arbor, MI: UMI Dissertation Services, ProQuest Information and Learning.

SECTION I

INTRODUCTION

1. Masten, J. E. (2007) *Aging with HIV/AIDS: The Experience of Gay Men in Late Middle Age*. Ann Arbor, MI: UMI Dissertation Services, ProQuest Information and Learning.

CHAPTER 1

1. Sondheim, S., & Goldman, J. (2001). *Follies* (Playwrights Canada Press). New York: Theatre Communications Group.

2. Davies, M. L. (1997). Shattered asssumptions: Time and the experience of long-term HIV-positivity. *Social Science and Medicine, 44*(5), 51–57.

3. Bury, M., & Holme, A. (1990). Quality of life and social support in the very old. *Journal of Aging Studies, 4*(4), 345–357; Strauss, A. (1987). *Qualitative Analysis for Social Scientists.* Cambridge, UK: University of Cambridge Press.

4. Charmaz, K. (1997). Identity dilemmas of chronically ill men. In A. Strauss & J. Corbin (Eds.), *Grounded Theory in Practice.* London, UK: Sage Publications; Charmaz, K. (2000). Experiencing chronic illness. In G. Albrecht, R. Fitzpatrick, & S. Scrimshaw (Eds.), *The Handbook of Social Studies in Health and Medicine.* London, UK: Sage Publications.

5. Moscowitz, J. T., & Wrubel, J. (2005). Coping with HIV as a chronic illness: A longitudinal analysis of illness appraisals. *Psychology and Health, August, 20*(4), 509–531.

6. Mitchell, C. G., & Linsk, N. L. (2004). A multidimensional conceptual framework for understanding HIV/AIDS as a chronic long-term illness. *Social Work, 49*(3), 469–478.

7. Nokes, K. M., Chew, L., & Altman, C. (2003). Using a telephone support group for HIV-positive persons aged 50+ to increase social support and health-related knowledge. *AIDS Patient Care and STDs, 17*(7), 345–351; Heckman, T., Barcikowski, R., Ogles, B., Suhr, J., Carlson, B., Holroyd, K., & Garske, J. (2006). A telephone-delivered coping improvement group intervention for middle-aged and older adults living with HIV/AIDS. *Annals of Behavioral Medicine, 32*(1), 27–38.

8. Robinson, W. A., Petty, Mary S., Patton, Cindy, & Kang, Helen. (2008). Aging with HIV: Historical and intra-community differences in experience of aging with HIV. *Journal of Gay and Lesbian Social Services, 20*(1), 127.

9. Marion, M. (1996). Living in an era of multiple loss and trauma: Understanding global loss in the gay community. In C. Alexander (Ed.), *Gay and Lesbian Mental Health.* New York: Harrington Park Press, p. 80.

CHAPTER 2

1. Gebo, K. A. (2006). HIV and aging: Implications for patient management. *Drugs & Aging, 23*(11), 897–913.

2. Jain, C. L., & Casau-Schulhof, N. (2009). HIV and the older adult. www.UpToDate.com.

3. Bhaskaran, K., Hamouda, O., Sannes M., *et al.* (2008). Changes in the risk of death after HIV seroconversion compared with mortality in the general population. *JAMA, 300,* 51.

4. Centers for Disease Control and Prevention. (2007). *HIV/AIDS Surveillance Report,* Vol. 19. Atlanta: U.S. Department of Health and Human Services, Centers for Disease Control and Prevention, 2009, 30. www.cdc.gov/hiv/topics/surrveillance/resources/reports.

5. Jain, C. L., & Casau-Schulhof, N. (2009). HIV and the older adult. www.UpToDate.com 2009.

6. Perez, J. L., & Moore, R.D. (2003). Greater effect of highly active antiretroviral therapy on survival in people aged 50 years compared with younger people in an urban observational cohort. *Clinical Infectious Disease, 36,* 212.

7. Grabar, S., Kousignian, I., Sobel, A., *et al.* (2004). Immunologic and clinical responses to highly active antiretroviral therapy over 50 years of age. Results from the French Hospital Database on HIV. *AIDS, 18,* 2029; Tumbarello, M., Rabagliati, R., de Gaetano, D. K., *et al.* (2004). Older age does not infuence CD4 cell recovery in HIV-1 infected patients receiving highly active antiretroviral therapy. *BMC Infectious Disease, 4,* 46; Viard, J. P., Mocroft, A., Chiesi, A., *et al.* Influence of age on CD4 cell recovery in human immunodeficiency virus—infected patients receiving highly active antiretroviral therapy: Evidence from EuroSida study. *Journal of Infectious Disease, 183,* 1290.

8. Lodwick, R. K., Smith, C. J., Youle, M., *et al.* (2008). Stability of antiretroviral regimens in patients with viral suppression. *AIDS, 22,* 1039; Sotaniemi, E. A., Arranto, A. J., Pelkonen, O., & Pasanen, M. (1997). Age and cytochrome P450-linked drug metabolism in humans: An analysis of 226 subjects with equal histopathologic conditions. *Clinical Pharmacology Therapies, 61,* 331; Knobel, H., Guelar, A., Valldecillo, G., *et al.* (2001). Response to highly active antiretroviral therapy in HIV-infected patients aged 60 years or older after 24 months follow-up. *AIDS, 15,* 1591.

9. Jain, C. L., & Casau-Schulhof, N. (2009). HIV and the older adult. www.UpToDate.com; Aberg, J. A., Kaplan, J. E., Libman, H., *et al.* Primary care guidelines for the management of persons infected with human immunodeficiency virus: 2009 update by the HIV Medicine Association of the Infectious Disease Society of America. *Clinical Infectious Disease, 49,* 651–681; Dube, M. P., Stein, J. H., Aberg, J. A., *et al.* (2003). Guidelines for the evaluation and management of dyslipidemia in human immunodeficiency virus (HIV)-infected adults receiving antiretroviral therapy: Recommendations of the HIV Medicine Association of the Infectious Disease Society of America and the Adult AIDS Clinical Trials Group. *Clinical Infectious Disease, 37,* 613–627.

10. Wolfe, D. (2000). *Men Like Us: GMHC Guide to Gay Men's Sexual, Physical and Emotional Well Being.* New York: Ballantine Books.

11. Vaillant, G. E. (2002). *Aging Well: Surprising Guideposts to a Happier Life from the Landmark Harvard Study of Adult Development*. Boston: Little, Brown & Co.

12. *Physicians' Desk Reference* (58th ed.). (2004). Montvale, NJ: Thomson PDR.

13. Dixon, R. A., DeFrias, C. M., & Maitland, S. B. (2001). Memory in midlife. In M. Lachmen (Ed.), *The Handbook of Midlife Development* (pp. 248–278). New York: Wiley Publications.

14. Saxon, S. V., & Etten, M. J. (2002). *Physical Change & Aging: A Guide for the Helping Professions* (4th ed.). New York: The Tiresias Press, Inc.

15. Valcour, V., Shikuma, C., Shiramizu, B., *et al.* (2004). Higher frequency of dementia in older HIV-1 individuals. The Hawaii Aging with HIV-1 Cohort. *Neurology, 63,* 822; Vance D. E., & Robinson, F. P. (2004). Reconciling successful aging with HIV: A biopsychosocial overview. In C. C. Poindexter & S. Keigher (Eds.), *Midlife and Older Adults and HIV: Implications for Social Service Research, Practice and Policy* (pp. 59–78). New York: Haworth Press; Neundorfer, M. M., Camp, C. J., Lee, M. M., Skranjer, M. J., Malone, M. L., & Carr, J. R. (2004). Compensating for cognitive deficits in persons aged 50 and over with HIV/AIDS: A pilot study of a cognitive intervention. In C. Poindexter & S. Keigher (Eds.), *Midlife and Older Adults and HIV: Implications for Social Service Research, Practice and Policy*. New York: Haworth Press; Cherner, M., Ellis, R., Lazzaretto, D., Young, C., Mindt, M., Atkinson, J., Grant, I., Heaton, R., & HNRC Group. (2004). Effects of HIV-1 infection and aging on neurobehavioral functioning: Preliminary finding. *AIDS, 18*(Suppl 1), S27–S34; Becker, J. T., Lopez, O. L., Dew, M. A., & Aizenstein, H. J. (2004). Prevalence of cognitive disorders differs as a function of age in HIV virus infection. *AIDS, 18*(Suppl 1), S11–S18.

16. Ances, B. M., *et al.* (2010). HIV and aging independently affect brain function as measured by functional magnetic resonance imaging. *Journal of Infectious Diseases, 201,* 336–340.

17. Ettenbofer, M. L., Hinkin, C. H., Castellon, S. A., Durvasula, R., Uliman, J., Lam, M., Myers, H., Wright, M. J., & Foley, J. (2009). Aging, neurocognition, and medication adherence in HIV infection. *American Journal of Geriatric Psychiatry, 17*(4), 281–290; Vance, D. E., Struzick, T. C., & Masten, J. (2008). Hardiness, successful aging, and HIV: implications for social work. *Journal of Gerontological Social Work, 51,* 260–283.

18. Weil, A. (2005). *Healthy Aging: A Lifelong Guide to Your Well-Being.* New York: Anchor Books.

19. Saxon, S. V., & Etten, M. J. (2002). *Physical Change & Aging: A Guide for the Helping Professions* (4th ed.). New York: The Tiresias Press, Inc.;

Katchadurian, H. A. (1987). *Fifty Midlife in Perspective.* New York: W.H. Freeman; Bergquist, W. H., Greenberg, E. M., & Klaum, G. A. (Eds.). (1993). *In Our Fifties.* San Francisco: Jossey-Bass; Willis, S. L., & Reid, J. D. (Eds). (1999). *Life in the Middle: Psychological and Social Development in Middle Age.* New York: Academic Press.

20. Linsk, N. L. (1997). Experience of older gay and bisexual men living with HIV/AIDS. *Journal of Gay, Lesbian and Bisexual Identity, 2*(3/4); Siegel, K., Dean, L., & Schrimshaw, E. W. (1999). Symptom ambiguity among late-middle-age and older adults with HIV. *Research on Aging, 21*(4), 595–618.

CHAPTER 3

1. Rowe, J. W., & Kahn, R. L. (1998). *Successful Aging.* New York: Dell Publishing.

2. Quam, J. K., & Whitford, G. S. (1992). Adaptation and age-related expectations of older gay and lesbian adults. *The Gerontologist, 32,* 367–374; Dorfman, R., Wlters K., Burke, P., Hardin, L., Karanik, T., Raphael, J., & Silverstein, E. (1995). Old, sad and alone: The myth of the aging homosexual. *Journal of Gerontological Social Work, 24*(1–2), 29–35; Grossman, A., D'Augelli, A. R., & Herschberger, S. (2000). Social support networks of lesbian, gay and bisexual adults 60 years of age and older. *Journal of Gerontology, 55*(3), 171–179.

3. Emlet, C. A. (1993). Service utilization among older people with AIDS: Implications for case management. *Journal of Case Management, 2*(4), 119–124; Swindells, S., Mohr, J., Justis, J. C., Berman, S., Squier, C., Wagener, M. M., & Singh, N. (1999). Quality of life in patients with human immunodeficiency virus infection: Impact of social support, coping style and hopelessness. *International Journal of STD & AIDS, 10*(6), 383–391; Nichols, J. E., Speer, D. C., Watson, B. J., Watson, M. R., Vergon, T. L., Valee, C. M., & Meah, J. M. (2002). *Aging with HIV: Psychological, Social, and Health Issues.* New York: Academic Press; Shippy R. A., & Karpiak, S. E. (2005). Perceptions of support among older adults with HIV. *Research on Aging, 73*(3), 290–306.

4. Schrimshaw, E. W., & Siegel, K. (2003). Perceived barriers to social support from family and friends among older adults with HIV/AIDS. *Journal of Health Psychology, 8*(6), 738–752.

5. Bergquist,W. H., Greenberg, E. M., & Klaum, G. A. (Eds.). (1993). *In Our Fifties.* San Francisco: Jossey-Bass; Hunter, S., & Sundel, M. (1989). *Midlife Myths: Issues, Feelings, and Practice Applications.* Newbury Park, CA: Sage Publications.

6. Heckman, T. G., Somlai, A. M., Kalichman, S. C., Franzoi, S. L., & Kelly, J A. (1998). Psychosocial differences between urban and rural people living with HIV/AIDS. *Journal of Rural Health, 14*(2), 138–145.

7. Nokes, K. M., Chew, L., & Altman, C. (2003). Using a telephone support group for HIV-positive persons aged 50+ to increase social support and health-related knowledge. *AIDS Patient Care and STDs, 17*(7), 345–351. Heckman, T., Barcikowski, R., Ogles, B., Suhr, J., Carlson, B., Holroyd, K., & Garske, J. (2007). A telephone-delivered coping improvement group intervention for middle-aged and older adults living with HIV/AIDS. *Annals of Behavioral Medicine, 11*, 5–14.

8. Rowe, J. W., & Kahn, R. L. (1998). *Successful Aging.* New York: Dell Publishing.

9. Emlet, C. A. (1993). Service utilization among older people with AIDS: Implications for case management. *Journal of Case Management, 2*(4), 119–124; Linsk, N. L. (1997). Experience of older gay and bisexual men living with HIV/AIDS. *Journal of Gay, Lesbian and Bisexual Identity, 2*(3/4); Kalichman, S. C., Heckman, T., Kochman, A., Sikkema, K., & Bergholte, J. (2000). Depression and thoughts of suicide among middle aged and older persons living with HIV/AIDS. *Psychiatric Services, 51*(7), 903–907.

10. Chesney, M. A., Chambers, D. B., Taylor, J. M., & Johnson, L. M. (2003). Social support, distress, and well-being in older men living with HIV infection. *JAIDS, 33*, S185–S193.

CHAPTER 4

1. Quarto, J. (1997). Aging in the midst of AIDS: Perspectives on the elderly gay male in the 1990s. In L. B. Brown, S. G. Sarosy, T. C. Cook, & J. G. Quarto, (Eds.), *Gay Men and Aging.* New York: Garland Publications.

2. www.lambdalegal.org

3. D'Augelli, A., & Grossman, A. (2001). Aspects of mental health among older lesbian, gay and bisexual adults. *Aging and Mental Health, 5*(2), 149–158.

4. Linsk, N. L. (1997). Experience of older gay and bisexual men living with HIV/AIDS. *Journal of Gay, Lesbian and Bisexual Identity, 2*(3/4); Nichols, J. E., Speer, D. C., Watson, B. J., Watson, M. R., Vergon, T. L., Valee, C. M., & Meah, J. M. (2002). *Aging with HIV: Psychological, Social, and Health Issues.* New York: Academic Press; Siegel, K., & Schrimshaw, E. W. (2003). Reasons for the adoption of celibacy among older men and women living with HIV/AIDS. *Journal of Sex Research, 40*(2), 189–200.

5. Brown, D. R., & Sankar, A. (1998). HIV/AIDS and aging minority populations. *Research on Aging, 20*(6), 865–884, p. 865.

6. Speer, D. C., Kennedy, M., Watson, M., Meah, J., Nichols, J., & Watson, B. (1999). Ethnic, demographic and social differences among middle aged and older adults with HIV/AIDS. *AIDS Patients Care and STDs, 13*(10), 615–624.

CHAPTER 5

1. Bergquist, W. H., Greenberg, E. M., & Klaum, G. A. (Eds.). (1993). *In Our Fifties*. San Francisco: Jossey-Bass; Hunter, S., & Sundel, M. (1989). *Midlife Myths: Issues, Feelings, and Practice Applications*. Newbury Park, CA: Sage Publications; Willis, S. L., & Reid, J. D. (Eds.). (1999). *Life in the Middle: Psychological and Social Development in Middle Age*. New York: Academic Press; Weg, R. (1989). Biology and physiology of development of aging. *Gerontology and Geriatrics Education*, 9(4), 9–16.

2. Wolfe, D. (2000). *Men Like Us: GMHC Guide to Gay Men's Sexual, Physical and Emotional Well Being*. New York: Ballantine Books.

3. Nichols, J. E., Siegel, K., & Schrimshaw, E. W. (2003). Reasons for the adoption of celibacy among older men and women living with HIV/AIDS. *Journal of Sex Research*, 40(2), 189–200.

4. SCA Publication No. SCA-001, 1995.

5. Carnes, P. (1992). *Don't Call It Love: Recovery from Sexual Addiction*. New York: Bantam Books. P. 314.

CHAPTER 6

1. Erikson, E. H. (1963). *Childhood and Society*. New York: W. W. Norton and Company; Goldstein, E. G. (1997). *Ego Psychology and Social Work Practice*. New York: The Free Press.

2. Vaillant, G. E. (2002). *Aging Well: Surprising Guideposts to a Happier Life from the Landmark Harvard Study of Adult Development*. Boston: Little, Brown and Co., p. 100.

3. Hass, M. (2002). Social support as relationship maintenance in gay male couples coping with HIV or AIDS. *Journal of Social and Personal Relationships*, 19(1), 87–111; Brown, L. B., Sarosy, S. G., Cook, T. C., & Quarto, J. G. (2001). *Gay Men and Aging*. New York: Garland Publications; Cruz, M. J. (2004). *Sociological Analysis of Aging: The Gay Male Perspective*. New York: Harrington Park Press.

4. Barusch, A. S. (2008). *Love Stories of Later Life: A Narrative Approach to Understanding Romance*. New York: Oxford University Press.

5. Vaillant, G. E. (2002). *Aging Well: Surprising Guideposts to a Happier Life from the Landmark Harvard Study of Adult Development*. Boston: Little, Brown & Co., p. 46.

CHAPTER 7

1. Willis S. L., & Reid, J. D. (Eds.). (1999). *Life in the Middle: Psychological and Social Development in Middle Age*. New York: Academic Press.

2. Aron, L. (1996). *A Meeting of Minds: Mutuality in Psychoanalysis.* Hillsdale, NJ: The Analytic Press; Beebe, B., & Lachmann, F. M. (1988). The contribution of mother-infant mutual influence to the origins of self-esteem and object representations. *Psychoanalytic Psychology, 5,* 305–337; Benjamin, J. (1990). An outline in intersubjectivity: The development of recognition. *Psychoanalytic Psychology, 7,* 33–46; Stern, D. (1985). *The Interpersonal World of the Infant: A View from Psychoanalysis and Developmental Psychology.* New York: Basic Books; Winnicott, D. H. (1965). *Maturational Processes.* London, UK: Tavistock Publications.

3. Erikson, E. H. (1963). *Childhood and Society.* New York: W. W. Norton and Company; Greenberg, J. R., & Mitchell, S. A. (1983). *Object Relations in Psychoanalytic Theory.* Cambridge, MA: Harvard University Press.

4. Vaillant, G. E. (2002). *Aging Well: Surprising Guideposts to a Happier Life from the Landmark Harvard Study of Adult Development.* Boston: Little, Brown & Co.

5. McGoldrick, M., & Gerson, R. (1985). *Genograms in Family Assessment.* New York: W.W. Norton and Company.

6. Shippy R. A., & Karpiak, S. E. (2005). Perceptions of support among older adults with HIV. *Research on Aging, 73*(3), 290–306.

CHAPTER 8

1. Erikson, E. H. (1963). *Childhood and Society.* New York: W.W. Norton and Company, p. 266.

2. Tamir, L. M. (1982). *Men in the Forties: The Transition to Middle Age.* New York: Springer Publications

3. Farrell, M. P., & Rosenberg, S. D. (1981). *Men at Midlife.* Boston, MA: Auburn House.

4. Levinson, D. (1978). *The Seasons of a Man's Life.* New York: Alfred A. Knopf.

5. Vaillant, G. E. (2002). *Aging Well: Surprising Guideposts to a Happier Life from the Landmark Harvard Study of Adult Development.* Boston: Little, Brown & Co.

6. Ellis, A. (2001). *Gay Men at Midlife: Age before Beauty.* Binghamton, NY: Harrington Park Press; Peacock, J. R. (2000). Gay male adult development: Some stage issues for an older cohort. *Journal of Homosexuality, 40*(2), 13–29; Adelman, M. (1990). Stigma, gay lifestyles and adjustment to aging: A study of later-life gay men and lesbians. *Journal of Homosexuality, 20*(2–4), 7–32.

7. Vaillant, G. E. (2002) *Aging Well: Surprising Guideposts to a Happier Life from the Landmark Harvard Study of Adult Development.* Boston: Little, Brown & Co.

8. Berguist, W. H., Greenberg, E. M., & Klaum, G. A. (Eds.). (1993). *In Our Fifties.* San Francisco: Jossey-Bass, p. 487.

9. Vaillant, G. E. (2002). *Aging Well: Surprising Guideposts to a Happier Life from the Landmark Harvard Study of Adult Development.* Boston: Little, Brown & Co., p. 224.

CHAPTER 9

1. Vaillant, G. E. (2002). *Aging Well: Surprising Guideposts to a Happier Life from the Landmark Harvard Study of Adult Development.* Boston: Little, Brown & Co.

2. Erikson, E. H. (1963). *Childhood and Society.* New York: W.W. Norton and Company, Inc.; Greenberg, J. R., & Mitchell, S. A. (1983). *Object Relations in Psychoanalytic Theory.* Cambridge, MA: Harvard University Press; Vaillant, George E. (2002). *Aging Well: Surprising Guideposts to a Happier Life from the Landmark Harvard Study of Adult Development.* Boston: Little, Brown & Co.

3. Kimmel, D. C. (1980). *Adulthood and Aging: An Interdisciplinary, Developmental View.* New York: John Wiley & Sons.

4. Kertzner, R. M., & Sved, M. (1996). Midlife gay men and lesbians: Adult development and mental health. In R. P. Cabaj & T. S. Stein (Eds.), *Textbook of Homosexuality and Mental Health.* Washington, DC: American Psychiatric Press, p. 289.

5. Siegel, K., Raveis, V., & Karus, D. (1998). Perceived advantages and disadvantages of age among older HIV-infected adults. *Research on Aging, 20*(6), 686–711, p. 707.

6. Barusch, A. S. (2008). *Love Stories of Later Life: A Narrative Approach to Understanding Romance.* New York: Oxford University Press; Carstensen, L. L., Pasupathi, M., Mayr, U., & Nesselroade, J. R. (1998). Emotional experience in everyday life across the adult life span. *Journal of Personality and Social Psychology, 79,* 644–655; Birditt, K. S., & Fingerman, L. L. (2005). Do we get better at picking our battles? Age group differences in descriptions of behavioral reactions to interpersonal tensions. *Journal of Gerontology: Psychological Sciences, 60B*(3), 121–138.

7. Vaillant, G. E. (2002). *Aging Well: Surprising Guideposts to a Happier Life from the Landmark Harvard Study of Adult Development.* Boston: Little, Brown & Co.

8. Nichols, J. E., Speer, D. C., Watson, B. J., Watson, M. R., Vergon, T. L., Valee, C. M., & Meah, J. M. (2002). *Aging with HIV: Psychological, Social, and Health Issues.* New York: Academic Press.

9. Heckman, T., Kochman, A., & Sikkema, K. (2002). Depressive symptoms in older adults living with HIV disease: Application of the chronic illness quality of life model. *Journal of Mental Health and Aging, 8*(4), 267–286.

SECTION II

INTRODUCTION

1. Erikson, E. H. (1963). *Childhood and Society*. New York: W. W. Norton and Company, Inc.; Greenberg, J. R., & Mitchell, S. A. (1983). *Object Relations in Psychoanalytic Theory*. Cambridge, MA: Harvard University Press.

2. Masten, J. E. (2007). *Aging with HIV/AIDS: The Experience of Gay Men in Late Middle Age*. Ann Arbor, MI: UMI Dissertation Services, ProQuest Information and Learning.

3. The questions posed are not intended to be an exhaustive exploration of adaptation and stagnation. Instead, they present the subtle, and often difficult to discern differences between the two. Each question contains two codes from the research data. When positioned next to each other, they offer the reader an opportunity to reevaluate his subjective experience and determine for himself whether his choices are adaptive or represent stagnation in his process of aging with HIV.

CHAPTER 10

1. Yep, G. A., Lovaas, K. E., & Pagonis, A. V. (2002). The case of 'riding bareback': Sexual practices and the paradoxes of identity in the era of AIDS. *Journal of Homosexuality, 42*(4), 1–14.

2. Charmaz, K. (1997). Identity dilemmas of chronically ill men. In A. Strauss & J. Corbin (Eds.), *Grounded Theory in Practice*. London, UK: Sage Publications, p. 229.

3. Bluck, S., & Alea, N. (2002). Exploring the functions of autobiographical memory: Why do I remember the autumn? In J. D. Webster & B. K. Haight (Eds.), *Critical Advances in Reminiscence Work: From Theory to Application* (pp. 61–75). New York: Springer Publishing Company; Cappeliez, P., O'Rourke, N., & Chaudhury, H. (2005). Functions of reminiscence and mental health in later life. *Aging & Mental Health, 9*(4), 295–301.

CHAPTER 11

1. Joyce, G. F., Goldman, D. P., Leibowitz, A. A., Alpert, A., & Bao, Y. (2005). A socioeconomic profile of older adults with HIV. *Journal of Health Care for the Poor and Underserved, 16*(1), 12–28.

2. Kalichman, S. C., Heckman, T., Kochman, A, Sikkema, K., & Bergholte, J. (2000). Depression and thoughts of suicide among middle aged and older persons living with HIV/AIDS. *Psychiatric Services, 51*(7), 903–907; Nichols, J. E., Speer, D. C., Watson, B. J., Watson, M. R., Vergon, T. L., Valee, C. M., &

Meah, J. M. (2002). *Aging with HIV: Psychological, Social, and Health Issues.* New York: Academic Press.

3. Emlet, C. A. (1993). Service utilization among older people with AIDS: Implications for case management. *Journal of Case Management, 2*(4), 119–124; Linsk, N. L. (1997). Experience of older gay and bisexual men living with HIV/AIDS. *Journal of Gay, Lesbian and Bisexual Identity, 2*(3/4); Shippy R. A., & Karpiak, S. E. (2005). The aging HIV/AIDS population: Fragile social networks. *Aging and Mental Health, 9*(3), 246–254; Shulman, Lawrence. (1992). *The Skills of Helping Individuals, Families, and Groups* (3rd ed.). Itasca, IL: F. E. Peacock Publishers, Inc.; Nichols, J. E., Speer, D. C., Watson, B. J., Watson, M. R., Vergon, T. L., Valee, C. M., & Meah, J. M. (2002). *Aging with HIV: Psychological, Social, and Health Issues.* New York: Academic Press.

4. Poindexter, C. P., & Shippy, A. R. (2008). Networks of older New Yorkers with HIV: Fragility, resilience, and transformation. *AIDS Patient Care and STDs, 22*(9), 723–733.

5. Heckhausen, J. (2001). Adaptation and resilience in midlife. In M. Lachmen, *The Handbook of Midlife Development* (pp. 345–395). New York: John Wiley Publications.

6. Penrod, J., Gueldner, S. H., & Poon, L. W. (2003). Managing multiple chronic health conditions in everyday life. In L. W. Poon, S. H. Gueldner, & B. Sprouse (Eds.), *Successful Aging and Adaptations with Chronic Diseases.* New York: Springer Publishing Company.

7. Alcoholics Anonymous World Services, Inc. (2003). *Twelve Steps and Twelve Traditions.* New York: Alcoholics Anonymous World Services, Inc., p. 41.

CHAPTER 12

1. Charmaz, K. (1997). Identity dilemmas of chronically ill men. In A. Strauss & J. Corbin (Eds.), *Grounded Theory in Practice.* London, UK: Sage Publications, p. 47.

2. Erikson, E. H. (1963). *Childhood and Society.* New York: W. W. Norton and Company, Inc.; Greenberg, J. R., & Mitchell, S. A. (1983). *Object Relations in Psychoanalytic Theory.* Cambridge, MA: Harvard University Press.

3. Vaillant, G. E. (2002). *Aging Well: Surprising Guideposts to a Happier Life from the Landmark Harvard Study of Adult Development.* Boston: Little, Brown & Co., p. 53.

CHAPTER 13

1. Alcoholics Anonymous World Services, Inc. (1998). *Living Sober.* New York: Alcoholics Anonymous World Services, Inc., p. 7.

2. Vaillant, G. E. (2002). *Aging Well: Surprising Guideposts to a Happier Life from the Landmark Harvard Study of Adult Development*. Boston: Little, Brown & Co., p. 308.

SECTION III

INTRODUCTION

1. Masten, J. E. (2007). *Aging with HIV/AIDS: The Experience of Gay Men in Late Middle Age*. Ann Arbor, MI: UMI Dissertation Services, ProQuest Information and Learning.

STEP 1

1. Vance D. E., & Robinson, F. P. (2004). Reconciling successful aging with HIV: A biopsychosocial overview. In C. C. Poindexter & S. Keigher (Eds.), *Midlife and Older Adults and HIV: Implications for Social Service Research, Practice and Policy* (pp. 59–78). New York: Haworth Press.

2. Panel on Antiretroviral Guidelines for Adults and Adolescents. Guidelines for the use of antiretroviral agents in HIV-1-infected adults and adolescents. Department of Health and Human Services. December 1, 2009, 1–161. Available at www.aidsinfo.nih.gov/ContentFiles/AdultandAdolescentGL .pdf.

3. *Ibid.*

4. Lee, S. D. (2008). *HIV and Aging* (pp. 64–65). New York: Informa Healthcare USA.

5. Aberg, J. A. (2009). Primary care guidelines for the management of persons infected with human immunodeficiency virus: 2009 update by the HIV Medicine Association of the Infectious Diseases Society of America. *Clinical Infectious Diseases, 49*, 676–678.

6. Panel on Antiretroviral Guidelines for Adults and Adolescents. (2009). Guidelines for the use of antiretroviral agents in HIV-1-infected adults and adolescents. Department of Health and Human Services. December 1, 2009, 1–161. Available at http://www.aidsinfo.nih.gov/ContentFiles/ AdultandAdolescentGL.pdf.

7. *Ibid.*

8. Rowe, J. W., & Kahn, R. L. (1998). *Successful Aging*. New York: Dell Publishing.

9. Vance, D. E., Ross, L. A., & Downs, C. A. (2009). Self-reported cognitive ability and global cognitive performance in adults with HIV. *Journal of Neuroscience Nursing, 40*(1), 6–13.

10. Lee, S. D. (2008). *HIV and Aging* (pp. 91–99). New York: Informa Healthcare USA.

11. Larson, E. B., Wang, L., Bowen, J. D., McCormick, W. C., Teri, L., Crane, P., & Kukull, W. (2006). Exercise is associated with reduced risk for incident dementia among persons 65 years of age and older. *Annals of Internal Medicine, 144*, 73–81.

STEP 2

1. Vaillant, G. E. (2002). *Aging Well: Surprising Guideposts to a Happier Life from the Landmark Harvard Study of Adult Development*. Boston: Little, Brown & Co.

STEP 3

1. Erikson, E. H. (1963). *Childhood and Society*. New York: W.W. Norton and Company, Inc.; Greenberg, J. R., & Mitchell, S. A. (1983). *Object Relations in Psychoanalytic Theory*. Cambridge, MA: Harvard University Press, p. 266.
2. Kimmel, D. C. (1980). *Adulthood and Aging: An Interdisciplinary, Developmental View*. New York: John Wiley & Sons.
3. Peacock, J. R. (2000). Gay male adult development: Some stage issues for an older cohort. *Journal of Homosexuality, 40*(2), 13–29.

STEP 4

1. Gabriel, M. A. (1996). *AIDS Trauma and Support Group Therapy: Mutual Aid, Empowerment, Connection*. New York: The Free Press.
2. Alexander, R. A. (1987). The relationship between internalized homophobia and depression and low self-esteem in gay men. *Dissertation Abstracts International, 47*, 3977A; Dupras, A. (1994). Internalized homophobia and psychosexual adjustment among gay men. *Psychological Reports, 75*(1,1), 23–28; Nicholson, W. D., & Long, B. C. (1990). Self-esteem, social support, internalized homophobia, and coping strategies of HIV+ gay men. *Journal of Consulting and Clinical Psychology, 558*(6), 873–876.
3. Weil, A. (2005). *Healthy Aging: A Lifelong Guide to Your Well-Being*. New York: Anchor Books, p. 106.
4. Kimmel, D. C. (1980). *Adulthood and Gging: An Interdisciplinary, Developmental View*. New York: John Wiley & Sons, p. 117.

STEP 5

1. Kubler-Ross, E. (2005). *On Grief and Grieving: Finding the Meaning of Grief Through the Five Stages of Loss*. New York: Simon & Schuster Ltd.

2. Barusch, A. S. (2008). *Love Stories of Later Life: A Narrative Approach to Understanding Romance*. New York: Oxford University Press.

STEP 6

1. American Psychiatric Association. (2000). *Diagnostic and Statistical Manual of Mental Disorders* (4th ed., Text Revision). Washington, DC: American Psychiatric Association.

2. Vaillant, G. E. (2002). *Aging Well: Surprising Guideposts to a Happier Life from the Landmark Harvard Study of Adult Development*. Boston: Little, Brown & Co.

STEP 7

1. Vaillant, G. E. (2002). *Aging Well: Surprising Guideposts to a Happier Life from the Landmark Harvard Study of Adult Development*. Boston: Little, Brown & Co.

2. Heckman, T., Kochman, A., Sikkema, K. J., Kalichman, S. C., Masten, J., Bergholte, J., & Catz, S. (2001). A pilot coping improvement intervention for late middle aged and older adults living with HIV/AIDS in the USA. *AIDS, 13*(1), 129–139.

3. Lazarus, R. S., & Folkman, S. (1984). *Stress, Appraisal, and Coping*. New York: Springer Publishing.

STEP 8

1. Nichols, J. E., Speer, D. C., Watson, B. J., Watson, M. R., Vergon, T. L., Valee, C. M., & Meah, J. M. (2002). *Aging with HIV: Psychological, Social, and Health Issues*. New York: Academic Press; Bergquist, W. H., Greenberg, E. M., & Klaum, G. A. (Eds.). (1993). *In Our Fifties*. San Francisco: Jossey-Bass. Erikson, E. H. (1997). *The Life Cycle Completed*. New York: Norton Press.

2. Alcoholics Anonymous World Services, Inc. (1976). *Alcoholics Anonymous* (3rd ed.). New York: Alcoholics Anonymous World Services, Inc., p. 62.

3. Cameron, J. (1992). *The Artist's Way: A Spiritual Path to Higher Creativity*. New York: G.P. Putnam's Sons.

4. Singh, K. D. (1998). *The Grace in Dying: How We Are Transformed Spiritually As We Die*. San Francisco: Harper.

5. Gibran, K. (1983). *The Prophet*. New York: Alfred A. Knopf, p. 25.

6. Weil, A. (2005). *Healthy Aging: A Lifelong Guide to Your Well-Being*. New York: Anchor Books, p. 296.

7. Vaillant, G. E. (2002). *Aging Well*. New York: Little, Brown & Company.

8. Jung, C. (1960). *The Structure and Dynamics of the Psyche (Collected Works of C. G. Jung, Volume 8)*. Princeton, NJ: Princeton University Press.

9. Kabat-Zinn, J. (2005). *Wherever You Go There You Are: Mindfulness Meditation in Everyday Life*. New York: Hyperion, p. 62.

10. Sri Swami Satchidananda. (1975). *Meditation*. Yogaville: Satchidananda Ashram.

STEP 9

1. Cameron, J. (1992). *The Artist's Way: A Spiritual Path to Higher Creativity*. New York: G.P. Putnam's Sons.

2. Orman, S. (2001). *The Road to Wealth: A Comprehensive Guide to Your Money*. New York: Riverhead Books, p. 190.

3. United States Department of Health and Human Services. (2009). www.medicare.gov/pdp-basic-information.asp.

ABOUT THE STUDY

1. NCHS Data Warehouse on Trends in Health and Aging. (2004). Trends in HIV/AIDS in aging Americans. www.cdc.gov/nchs/agingact.htm.

2. Justice, A. C. (1996). The role of functional status in predicting inpatient mortality with AIDS. *Journal of Clinical Epidemiology*, 49(2), 193–201; Chen, H. X., Ryan, P. A., Ferguson, R. P., Yataco, A., Markowitz, J. A., & Raksis, K. (1998). Characteristics of acquired immunodeficiency syndrome in older adults. *Journal of the American Geriatrics Society*, 46(2), 153–156.

3. Emlet, C. A., & Poindexter, C. C. (2004). Underserved, unseen and unheard: Integrating programs for HIV-infected and HIV-affect older adults. *Health and Social Work*, 29(2), 86–96; Kalichman, S. C., Heckman, T., Kochman, A., Sikkema, K., & Bergholte, J. (2000). Depression and thoughts of suicide among middle aged and older persons living with HIV/AIDS. *Psychiatric Services*, 51(7), 903–907; Swindells, S., Mohr, J., Justis, J. C., Berman, S., Squier, C., Wagener, M. M., & Singh, N. (1999). Quality of life in patients with human immunodeficiency virus infection: Impact of social support, coping style and hopelessness. *International Journal of STD & AIDS*, 10(6), 383–391; Shippy, R. A., & Karpiak, S. E. (2005). Perceptions of support among older adults with HIV. *Research on Aging*, 73(3), 290–306.

4. Siegel, K., Raveis, V., & Karus, D. (1998). Perceived advantages and disadvantages of age among older HIV-infected adults. *Research on Aging*, 20(6), 686–711.

5. Linsk, N. L. (1997). Experience of older gay and bisexual men living with HIV/AIDS. *Journal of Gay, Lesbian and Bisexual Identity*, 2(3/4).

6. Neugarten, B. L. (1986). *Middle Age and Aging: A Reader in Social Psychology*. Chicago: The University of Chicago Press.

7. Padgett, D. K. (1998). *Qualitative Methods in Social Work Research*. Thousand Oaks, CA: Sage Publications, p. 8.

8. Merriam, S. B. (2002). *Qualitative Research in Practice: Examples for Discussion and Analysis*. San Francisco, CA: Jossey-Bass, p. 38.

9. Padgett, D. K. (1998). *Qualitative Methods in Social Work Research*. Thousand Oaks, CA: Sage Publications, p. 2.

10. Charmaz, K. (2000). Experiencing chronic illness. In G. Albrecht, R. Fitzpatrick, & S. Scrimshaw (Eds.), *The Handbook of Social Studies in Health and Medicine*. London, UK: Sage Publication; Strauss, A. (1987). *Qualitative Analysis for Social Scientists*. Cambridge, UK: Cambridge University Press.

11. Rubin, A., & Babbie, E. (1997). *Research Methods for Social Work*. New York: Brook/Cole Publishing.

12. Muhr, T. (1997). *Atlas.ti: Visual Qualitative Data Analysis-Management Model Building–Release 4.1 User's Manual*. Berlin, Germany: Scientific Software Development.

13. Padgett, D. K. (1998). *Qualitative Methods in Social Work Research*. Thousand Oaks, CA: Sage Publications.

14. Aldwin, C. M., & Levenson, M. R. (2001). Stress, coping and health at midlife: A developmental perspective. In M. Lachmen (Ed.), *The Handbook of Midlife Development* (pp. 188–225). New York: John Wiley Publications; Berguist, W. H., Greenberg, E. M., & Klaum, G. A. (Eds.). (1993). *In Our Fifties*. San Francisco: Jossey-Bass. Farrell, M. P., & Rosenberg, S. D. (1981). *Men at Midlife*. Boston: Auburn House; Heckhausen, J. (2001). Adaptation and resilience in midlife. In M. Lachmen (Ed.), *The Handbook of Midlife Development* (pp. 345–395). New York: John Wiley Publications; Kertzner, R. M., & Sved, M. (1996). Midlife gay men and lesbians: Adult development and mental health. In R. P. Cabaj & T. S. Stein (Eds.), *Textbook of Homosexuality and Mental Health*. Washington, DC: American Psychiatric Press.

Index

Adaptation, 15, 22, 125, 207,
   215–218
  vs stagnation, theory of, 99–101, 125
Adult development, 56, 66, 76
  life stage model of, 87
Ageism, 42, 162–163
  internalized, 166
Agency, *see* Locus of control
Age-related diseases, 17–18
Aging, 35, 100
  immature defenses against, 178
  theories of, 56
Alcohol, 123, 144

Children, 65, 66, 73–74, 86
Cholesterol, 141
Cohort, *see* Peers
Coming out, *see* disclosure
Coping, 184
Creativity, *see* play
Crisis competence, 167

Death, fear of, 87
Defense mechanisms, *see* coping
Demographic characteristics, 69
Depression, 137, 176

Diabetes, 145
Diet and food, 144–145
Disability, 177
Disclosure, 38–39, 59
Doctors, 21–22, 139
Drugs, 19, 142, 143

Emotions, 91, 218
Erikson, Erik, 100, 157
Exercise, 146

Family, 65–68
Food, *see* diet and food
Friends, 50–52
  gain, 33–34
  loss, 12, 72

Gay community, 40–42
Gay identity, 55, 67
Generativity, 167–168
Grief, *see* loss

Health insurance, 197–198
Heart disease, 10
HIV
  infection, x, 9

HIV (*cont.*)
  medication, 22–23, 142
  psychological impact of-related
    health, 9
  stigma, 162–163
Homophobia, 161–162
  internalized, 162
Hypertension, 27, 28

Income, 76, 80, 196
Internet, 33, 34, 53, 152, 153
Intimacy, 56, 63, 64
Isolation, 33, 167

Learning, 81, 106, 203
Leisure, *see* play
Lipodystrophy, 24–25, 142
Living alone, 172
Locus of control, 114, 215
Loneliness, 23
Longitudinal study on aging, 84, 178
Long-term care, 198

MacArthur Foundation Study of
    Successful Aging, 143
Maturity, 88–91
Meditation, 185, 192
Memory loss, 26
Mental health, *see* psychological
    well-being
Mentoring, *see* volunteering
Mortality, 7, 9–10
  acceptance of, 14, 17
  "healthy denial," 127
  living/planning with, 125–126
  reflecting on, 72, 128
Multivitamins and supplements,
    146–147
Muscle mass, 144–145

Neuropathy, 17
Nutrition, *see* diet and food

Overweight, 179

Partnership status, *see* relationships
Personal control, *see* locus of control
Peer, ix, 30
Pet, 33, 63
Physical activity, *see* exercise
Play, 73, 203–205
Prayer, *see* spirituality
Preventive medicine, 140
Psychological well-being, 35,
    92, 114

Quality of life, 115

Racism, 44
Relationships
  intimate, 11, 56
  forming new relationships, 31
  loss, 35, 57
  long-term, 35, 57, 62
  short-term, 57
Relaxation techniques, 185–186
Religion, *see* spirituality
Remorse and regret, 106
Reminiscing, 106–107
Research
  on aging, 121, 154–155
  on aging with HIV, 155, 209–210
  on gay aging, 136
Resilience, 13, 155
Rest, *see* sleep
Retirement, 76, 79–80
Rewards of aging, 92, 117–118

Self-esteem, 42, 77, 167–168
Sex
  abstinence, 52
  activity, 38
  casual sex, 47
  compulsion, 53
  impotence, 50

in relationships, 40–41, 48
Sleep, 146
Smoking, 19, 143–144
Social network, *see* social support
Social support, 149–152
Socializing, 31, 203
Spirituality, 92–93
Stigma, 112–114, 161
Stress, 78, 103, 183
Successful aging model, 143
Supplements, *see* multivitamins and
    supplements
Survivor guilt, 12–13

"The look" of AIDS, 24, 68
Trauma, 7–9

Vaillant, George E., 57, 62, 66–67,
    84, 124, 184
Volunteering, 78, 154

Weil, Andrew, 148, 163, 168, 191
Work, 76–77

Yoga, 146